BLOCK CANCER NATURALLY

A 5-Pillar Guide to Prevent Cancer with Nutrition and Lifestyle Habits

C. Letitia Henry, DrPH, RDN

Disclaimer Notice

This book, authored by C. Letitia Henry, is intended for informational purposes only. It is not a substitute for professional medical advice, diagnosis, or treatment. She strongly advises readers to consult with their healthcare providers regarding the applicability of any aspects of the content to their own health and well-being.

If you have medical concerns, consult with your healthcare provider, physician, or another qualified medical professional.

© 2025 C. Letitia Henry - All rights reserved

No part of this book may be reproduced or transmitted in any form or by any means, electronic or mechanical, including photocopying, recording, or by any information storage and retrieval system, without written permission from the publisher.

What's Inside

About the Author...4

Introduction..5

The BLOCK Framework

- The BLOCK Analogy...8
- Building BLOCKs of Health.......................................14
    - Top 5 Cancer-Fighting Foods..............................15
    - Top 5 Nutritional Boosters...................................19
    - Top 5 Unhealthy Foods to Limit..........................23
    - Top 5 Cancer-Fighting Habits.............................27
    - Top 5 Cancer Risk Factors..................................31

Conclusion...35

Appendices..38

References...77

C. Letitia Henry, DrPH, RDN, CDCES, EP-C
Preventive Care Specialist

I'm Dr. Letitia Henry, a Preventive Care Specialist and the founder of The Prevention Specialists, LLC. With advanced credentials including a Doctorate in Public Health (DrPH), Registered Dietitian Nutritionist (RDN), Certified Diabetes Care and Education Specialist (CDCES), and Certified Exercise Physiologist (EP-C), I bring a wealth of expertise to the table. My goal is simple: to make healthier living achievable for everyone by breaking down complex health topics into clear, practical steps. I truly believe that prevention is the best medicine, and I'm dedicated to empowering you with knowledge and tools that support lasting lifestyle changes and better health outcomes.

My approach is rooted in simplicity and inclusivity, making it accessible for people from all backgrounds. I'm passionate about the idea that small, informed choices—like adding local, nutrient-rich foods to your meals—can lead to profound improvements in wellness and disease prevention. I aim to offer guidance and encouragement as you take steps toward better health.

In this book, I'm excited to share how everyday diet and lifestyle choices can strengthen your body's defenses against cancer and help you build a foundation for lifelong health. I look forward to joining you on this journey to a more empowered, healthier you.

Introduction

BLOCK Cancer Naturally

"Cancer prevention is a journey—each choice, each healthy habit, strengthens your body's defense, building a life that stands strong against cancer's reach." – C. Letitia Henry

Welcome to your guide to creating a lasting defense against cancer through intentional nutrition and lifestyle habits. Here, you'll explore the BLOCK framework—a set of five key pillars that strengthen your body's natural defenses. Preventing cancer takes more than one action; it's the combined impact of thoughtful choices that builds your body's strength and supports lifelong health.

Understanding how nutrition and lifestyle choices can prevent cancer starts with knowing what cancer is and how it develops. Cancer begins when cells grow and multiply uncontrollably. Normally, cells divide in an orderly way, replacing old or damaged ones. But cancer disrupts this cycle, causing damaged cells to multiply and form tumors that can spread throughout the body. It's not just one disease but a group of over 100 types that can affect nearly every organ, tissue, and bone. Common cancers include those of the breast, lung, skin, and colon, each sharing the same root cause: abnormal cell growth.

People have known about cancer for thousands of years, with mentions as early as ancient Egypt. But it wasn't until recent centuries that doctors began to understand how it spreads. Today, we know that daily lifestyle choices play a powerful role in either increasing or reducing our risk. By focusing on prevention, we can fortify the body's defenses and support its natural ability to repair and protect itself.

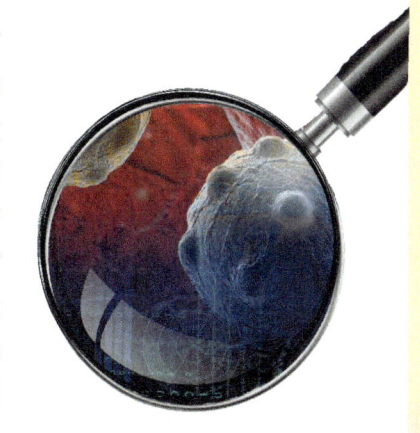

BLOCK Cancer Naturally

Each BLOCK pillar plays a unique role in supporting your health and creating a balanced approach to cancer prevention. The first pillar, **Boost Barrier**, enhances your antioxidant defenses against daily cell damage. **Lessen the Damage**, the second pillar, works to reduce inflammation in the body, which can cause harm over time if left unchecked. The third, **Oversee Repairs**, focuses on supporting DNA repair, so any minor cell damage can be fixed before it grows into a bigger issue. **Control Growth** regulates cell growth and enhances immune defense, keeping a close eye on abnormal cell changes. The final pillar, **Keep It Clean**, promotes gut health, helping the body clear out waste and stay balanced inside. Together, these pillars form a comprehensive approach to health, each reinforcing the others for maximum protection.

To get a clearer picture of where you currently stand, take a few minutes to complete the **BLOCK Self-Check in Appendix A**. This questionnaire will give insight into your habits, showing where you're already on track and highlighting areas that may need a little extra attention. This self-check can guide you as you go through the book, helping you see how each new choice makes a difference in your overall wellness.

The goal of this guide is to encourage small, manageable steps that lead to lasting change. Building a foundation of health doesn't mean overhauling everything at once. Instead, it's about starting where you are and making gradual shifts that are easy to maintain. Even adding one or two new habits at a time, like starting the day with a glass of water or adding leafy greens to your lunch, will add up to powerful benefits over time.

This book isn't just about information—it's packed with practical tools and resources, from recipes and shopping lists to guides on hydration, sleep, and stress relief. You'll find tips for healthy swaps,

BLOCK Cancer Naturally

exercise guides, and even support for quitting smoking. These resources are here to make healthy living simpler and help you build habits that last, so each step toward wellness feels natural.

As you begin this journey, think about your health goals and what matters most to you. Whether it's increasing energy, supporting immunity, or focusing on cancer prevention, remember that each small choice adds up to a stronger, healthier foundation. You have the power to take charge of your wellness through knowledge and proactive choices. Prevention is a powerful tool, and learning how each decision impacts your health is a step toward a more empowered, healthier you.

Now, let's dive into the BLOCK pillars and see how each one supports your body's foundation, working to reduce the risk of cancer. In the next section, we'll explore how these pillars work together to protect and strengthen your health into the future.

The BLOCK Analogy
Your Body is Like a House

"Building health is like building a strong house: each piece has a purpose, and together they create a foundation that stands against any storm." – C. Letitia Henry

Imagine your body as a house, where each BLOCK pillar acts as a structural element, keeping everything in balance and protected. Just like a house, your body relies on a solid foundation to weather life's storms. The nutrients you get from food and supplements are like bricks, beams, and paint, all working together to keep your "house" sturdy, clean, and resilient.

Think of each nutrient or healthy habit as a piece in a Jenga™ tower—adding strength and stability to the foundation. When you include foods rich in antioxidants, practice stress management, or stay active, you're adding "blocks" that reinforce your body's structure. But just as pulling out too many pieces from a Jenga tower can make it wobble and eventually fall, neglecting certain nutrients or lifestyle practices can weaken your health. Over time, this leaves your body more vulnerable to disease and damage.

By consistently reinforcing each BLOCK pillar with the right choices, you're helping to maintain a strong, balanced "house." Each pillar serves a purpose, creating a solid framework that empowers you to stay healthy and lower your risk of cancer. Let's explore each BLOCK pillar and see how they build a strong foundation for long-term wellness.

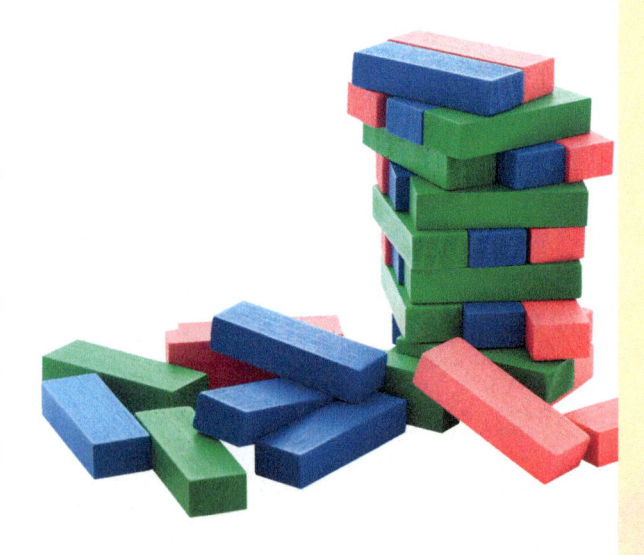

The BLOCK Analogy

B - Boost Barrier

"Just as paint shields a home from wear, antioxidants guard our cells, preserving strength from within." – C. Letitia Henry

Imagine an old house by the sea, where the sun, wind, and salty air have stripped away its protective paint over the years. Each time it rains, water seeps through the exposed concrete walls. The faded paint left the concrete vulnerable, allowing moisture to slip through the porous surface, gradually weakening the structure. Without a fresh layer of paint and sealant, the house grows more fragile with every storm.

Similarly, our bodies need consistent "barrier protection" to guard against daily wear and tear. Free radicals act like the relentless elements—sun, wind, and rain—gradually wearing down our cells. They enter the body through sources like UV rays, pollution, cigarette smoke, and even normal metabolism, causing tiny "cracks" over time. If these free radicals build up, they can damage cells and weaken your defenses.

Antioxidants act as a fresh "coat of paint" for your cells, helping to shield them from these free radicals. Foods rich in antioxidants, like berries, leafy greens, and cruciferous vegetables, build a strong defense, protecting cells from damage. Boosters like turmeric, green tea, garlic, ginger, and omega-3s add strength to this shield, while limiting processed foods and sugary snacks prevents extra strain on cells.

Habits like wearing sunscreen, staying hydrated, and avoiding smoke further protect your body, helping to keep your defenses strong over time.

Enhance Antioxidant Defense

The BLOCK Analogy
L - Lessen the Damage

"A single spark can bring down a house; controlling inflammation keeps the fire at bay." – C. Letitia Henry

Picture a kitchen where the stovetop flames have been left burning a little too long, sparking a small fire that scorches the cabinets and leaves smoke stains on the ceiling. But before it can spread, a quick-thinking firefighter neighbor rushes in and extinguishes the flames, stopping the fire in its tracks. The kitchen is saved from greater destruction, but the damage could have been severe if the fire hadn't been put out early.

In your body, inflammation acts much like that kitchen fire. It's helpful in small amounts, like when you get a cut or scrape, where inflammation rushes in to help healing. But when inflammation lingers or flares up repeatedly, it begins to act like a slow-burning fire, causing damage that gradually spreads throughout the body. Nutrients found in foods like berries, turmeric, and leafy greens are like firefighters, calming inflammation before it harms other tissues and becomes harder to control. Chronic inflammation, left unchecked, creates an environment where cancer cells can thrive, gradually weakening your "house."

Beyond diet, other habits help keep these "fires" under control. Regular exercise, managing stress, and getting enough sleep all act as extra "firefighters" alongside anti-inflammatory foods to keep your body balanced. Limiting items that fuel inflammation, like processed meats and fried foods, also helps maintain your body's "temperature." Together, these habits create a strong barrier against inflammation, promoting lasting health.

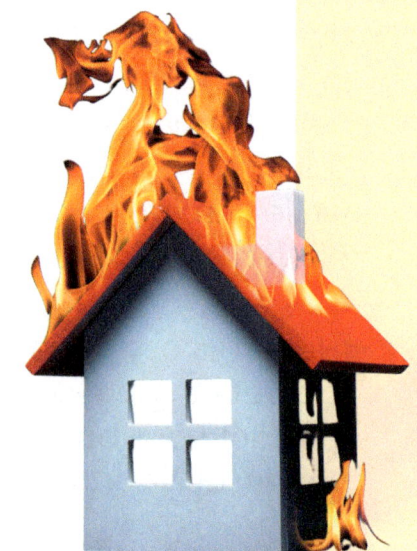

Reduce Inflammation

The BLOCK Analogy

O - Oversee Repairs

"Small cracks, if ignored, weaken the whole. DNA repair patches each fracture, reinforcing our foundation." – C. Letitia Henry

Consider a house that's been standing for years. Over time, tiny cracks start forming in the concrete foundation—not immediately noticeable, but they slowly weaken the stability of the house. If ignored, these small cracks widen, eventually threatening the entire structure. But with regular upkeep, skilled repair workers arrive to patch up each crack, strengthening the foundation and preventing further damage.

In your body, DNA repair functions much the same way, acting as that "repair team." Everyday exposures, like sunlight, environmental pollutants, or even natural aging, create tiny "cracks" in your DNA. If left unfixed, these can build up, leading to larger issues like cancer. Nutrients that support DNA repair, like folate, vitamin B12, and antioxidants, act like repair workers, finding and fixing small issues in cells to prevent them from becoming bigger problems.

And it's not just nutrients that support repairs—lifestyle habits like managing stress and getting enough sleep also strengthen your body's foundation by helping DNA repair. Limiting exposure to pollutants, radiation, and harmful chemicals reduces unnecessary damage, giving your cells a break from constant repair. Regular health screenings and knowing your family history allow for early detection, so preventive steps can be taken if needed. Together, these choices provide essential support, helping your body repair itself and stay strong over time.

Support DNA Repair

The BLOCK Analogy

C – Control Growth

"True wealth lies in safeguarding our health, just as a security system protects the heart of a home." – C. Letitia Henry

Picture stepping into a house equipped with a high-tech security system that monitors each entry and exit, making sure no unwanted guests slip in unnoticed. This system constantly scans for unusual activity, alerting the homeowners to any threats and providing peace of mind. In a similar way, your body relies on nutrients and healthy habits that work together to regulate cell growth and support immune function, acting as your internal security team. This system helps detect and remove abnormal cells before they become health threats like cancer.

Just as a security system has specific components that play different roles, nutrients like omega-3s, vitamin D, and zinc act as vigilant "guards" for your body, keeping the immune system alert. Found in foods like fatty fish, nuts, and seeds, omega-3s support immune health, while green tea and turmeric strengthen this defense, fostering balanced cell growth and healthy cellular function.

In addition to foods, lifestyle choices strengthen this security system. Physical activity supports immune health by helping remove harmful cells, while limiting red and processed meats reduces cancer risk. Regular screenings, like mammograms, and prostate checks, catch issues early, and understanding family cancer history—with genetic testing if needed— reinforces your defenses.

Together, these habits, proactive screenings, and supportive nutrients build a strong foundation, boosting this BLOCK pillar and promoting long-term health.

The BLOCK Analogy
K - Keep It Clean

"Clear pipes keep a house sound, and a balanced gut keeps the body thriving." – C. Letitia Henry

Envision a home with a carefully maintained plumbing system. Waste flows out smoothly, and clogs are rare because the pipes receive regular attention. Without this upkeep, toxins and waste would accumulate, causing blockages, odors, and even structural damage. Clean, well-maintained plumbing keeps the house fresh and livable.

In your body, supporting gut health is just as important. Fiber-rich foods, along with probiotics and prebiotics, act like the maintenance crew for your "plumbing," keeping everything moving efficiently and reducing toxin build-up. Staying hydrated is also essential, as water keeps things flowing smoothly, helping in natural detoxification. Exercise adds another layer of support, stimulating digestion and helping to prevent sluggishness or blockage in your system. Together, these practices keep your gut balanced and reduce inflammation, lowering your risk of harmful build-up.

Regular health screenings, like colonoscopies, are vital for early detection of potential issues in the intestines or colon, especially if there's a family history of colon cancer. By combining gut-friendly foods, hydration, active habits, and proactive screenings, you maintain a clean, healthy internal environment that supports long-term wellness.

With these pillars in place, let's move forward to explore in more detail the essential building blocks of health—foods, nutritional boosters, habits, and more—that work to reinforce your body's natural defenses.

Promote Gut Health

Building BLOCKs of Health
Five Core Practices

In the following sections, we'll explore five core practices within the BLOCK framework to guide you in preventing cancer naturally. Each core practice highlights specific foods, supplements, and health routines that fortify your body's defenses, helping you BLOCK cancer through intentional nutrition and lifestyle habits.

Top 5

Cancer-Fighting Foods: Discover nutrient-rich foods that serve as foundations for each BLOCK pillar.

Nutritional Boosters: Learn about powerful supplements and nutritional aids that enhance each BLOCK component.

Unhealthy Foods to Limit: Identify the foods that weaken each BLOCK pillar and understand how to limit their impact.

Cancer-Fighting Lifestyle Habits: Explore habits that support each BLOCK pillar, creating a solid foundation for health that extends beyond nutrition.

Cancer Risk Factors: Understand the key influences on cancer risk, from genetics to environmental exposures, helping you make informed, science-based choices for prevention.

These five core practices work to strengthen each BLOCK pillar, supporting your body's ability to build antioxidant defenses, reduce inflammation, repair DNA, control cell growth, and protect gut health. We'll start with the **Top 5 Cancer-Fighting Foods**, exploring nutrient-rich options that reinforce these pillars, creating a strong dietary base for cancer prevention.

TOP 5 Cancer-Fighting Foods

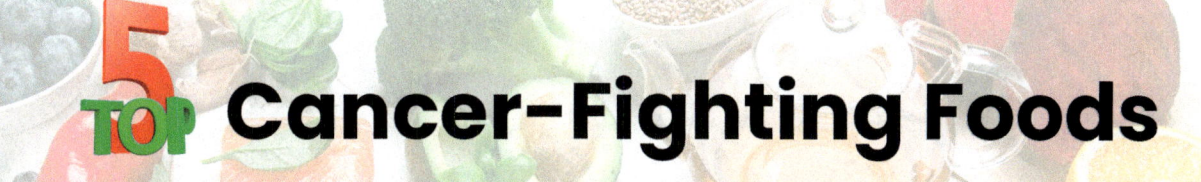

"A balanced plate is the first layer of protection—every color, every bite builds a stronger you." – C. Letitia Henry

A balanced, nutrient-rich diet is one of the strongest foundations for cancer prevention. Each food in your daily meals supports one or more BLOCK pillars—Boost Barrier, Lessen the Damage, Oversee Repairs, Control Growth, and Keep It Clean. In this section, we'll introduce five key foods aligned with each BLOCK category to help build a cancer-fighting diet.

For simplicity, each food appears under one pillar, though some offer multiple benefits. For example, berries are listed for Boost Barrier due to their antioxidants but also help reduce inflammation for Lessen the Damage. Think of these foods as essential 'building blocks' in your body's defenses, like structural elements in a well-built house.

1. Leafy Greens

- **Why They Matter:** Leafy greens, such as spinach, kale, collard greens, kallaloo greens (amaranth), and mustard greens, are packed with antioxidants, which protect your cells from free radicals—unstable molecules that can damage cells and lead to cancer. Think of these greens as the "paint" or protective coating on your house, shielding the exterior from weather and wear.
- **How Much:** Aim for 1 to 2 cups daily.
- **Simple Ways to Include Them:** Add a handful to smoothies, salads, or stir-fries, or use them as a base for wraps and bowls.

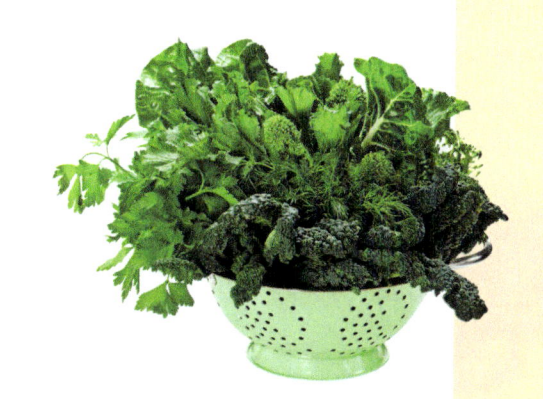

Foods for Defense

5 TOP Cancer-Fighting Foods

2. Berries

- **Why They Matter:** Berries, including blueberries, strawberries, blackberries, cranberries, and acerola cherries, contain powerful anti-inflammatory compounds that act like "firefighters" in your body, putting out inflammation before it spreads and causes further damage. Inflammation is a known risk factor for cancer, and these nutrients help keep it in check.
- **How Much:** Enjoy ½ cup of berries 3 to 4 times per week.
- **Simple Ways to Include Them:** Add to oatmeal, yogurt, or salads, or eat them on their own as a snack.

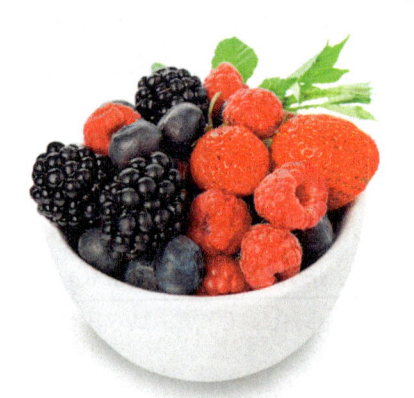

3. Cruciferous Vegetables

- **Why They Matter:** Cruciferous vegetables, such as broccoli, cauliflower, Brussels sprouts, cabbage, and bok choy, support the body's natural detoxification process and DNA repair. They're like skilled workers who patch up "cracks" in the foundation of your house, helping prevent long-term issues. By supporting DNA repair, these foods can help reduce the risk of cancerous mutations.
- **How Much:** Aim for at least 1 cup, 3 to 4 times a week.
- **Simple Ways to Include Them:** Roast, steam, or stir-fry these vegetables as a side dish or add them to soups and casseroles.

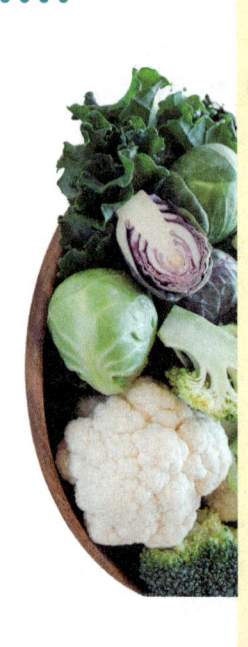

Foods for Defense

TOP 5 Cancer-Fighting Foods

4. Nuts and Seeds

- **Why They Matter:** Nuts and seeds, including walnuts, flaxseeds, chia seeds, Brazil nuts, and pumpkin seeds, are rich in healthy fats that help regulate cell growth and immune function. These healthy fats work like a well-maintained security system, ensuring that abnormal cells are detected and eliminated before they can cause harm.
- **How Much:** Enjoy a small handful (about ¼ cup) of nuts and seeds daily.
- **Simple Ways to Include Them:** Add to oatmeal, salads, or yogurt, or enjoy them as a snack on their own.

5. Beans and Legumes

- **Why They Matter:** Beans and legumes, like lentils, chickpeas, pigeon peas, black-eyed peas, and red kidney beans, are high in fiber, which supports gut health and digestion. Fiber acts like a well-maintained plumbing system, keeping waste flowing out and helping remove toxins from your body. A healthy gut reduces cancer risk by supporting internal balance.
- **How Much:** Aim for ½ cup of beans or legumes daily.
- **Simple Ways to Include Them:** Add to soups, salads, or grain bowls, or use them as a base for dips and spreads.

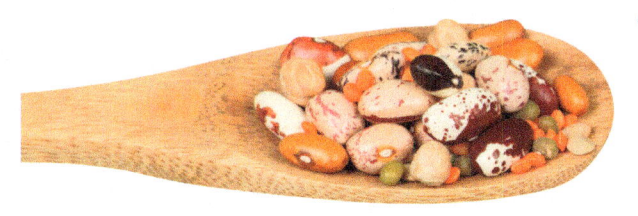

Foods for Defense

Top 5 Cancer-Fighting Foods

Including these top five foods in your weekly meal plan helps establish a solid foundation that strengthens each BLOCK pillar. Each food works with the others to create a balanced, cancer-preventive diet that fortifies your body's defenses from multiple angles. Consistency and variety are key—just as a well-built house relies on balanced support from each part of its structure.

Here's a sample menu that incorporates each BLOCK food group:
- **Breakfast:** Oatmeal with blueberries, chia seeds, and flaxseeds
- **Mid-Morning Snack**: Apple with almonds
- **Lunch:** Leafy green salad with spinach, kale, black beans, bell peppers, and cherry tomatoes, dressed with olive oil and lemon
- **Afternoon Snack:** Cucumber and carrot sticks with hummus
- **Dinner:** Grilled salmon with sautéed bok choy and steamed sweet potatoes

To create menus that suit your personal preferences, refer to the shopping list and recipes in **Appendix B**. These resources will help you develop meal plans that reinforce your health by supporting each BLOCK pillar and strengthening your body's defenses from all sides.

As you make these food choices, it's also essential to separate nutrition myths from facts. **Appendix C** provides more detail on common cancer nutrition myths, helping you make choices grounded in science. In the next section, we'll look at the **Top 5 Nutritional Boosters**—specific supplements and natural aids that offer added reinforcement for each category, ensuring your body has the resources it needs to stay strong. From antioxidants to immune-boosting nutrients, these boosters can be easily added to your routine, building on the foundation set by your diet.

Foods for Defense

Top 5 Nutritional Boosters

"Think of boosters as the fine-tuning tools in your diet, enhancing your body's natural defenses with each sip, sprinkle, and spoonful." – C. Letitia Henry

While some foods target specific health areas, certain nutritional boosters provide comprehensive support across all BLOCK pillars, acting like a true jack-of-all-trades that can handle every job needed to keep your body's 'house' in top shape. Listed in order of potency, turmeric, green tea, garlic, omega-3s, and ginger work beyond single purposes, delivering antioxidant protection, reducing inflammation, aiding DNA repair, regulating immune function, and supporting gut health.

These versatile boosters reinforce your body's defenses on all fronts, helping create a resilient, cancer-preventive foundation. Integrating these into your routine makes sure your health gains steady, balanced support, equipping your body with the resources to thrive.

1. Turmeric

- **Why It Matters:** Turmeric, with curcumin as its active ingredient, acts as a versatile defender. It targets inflammation, supports immunity, promotes cell repair, and aids digestion. Unlike foods that focus on one area, turmeric's broad effects reinforce each part of your body's defenses, creating a strong, layered shield for enhanced protection.
- **Recommended Amount:** 1/4 to 1/2 teaspoon of turmeric powder daily, or 500 to 1,000 mg of curcumin extract, both split into two doses.
- **Simple Ways to Include It:** Add turmeric powder to soups, curries, or smoothies, or consider a curcumin supplement for a concentrated dose.

TOP 5 Nutritional Boosters

2. Green Tea

- **Why It Matters:** Green tea is like a quality inspector, checking every part of your body's structure to make sure nothing slips through the cracks. The catechins in green tea, particularly EGCG (Epigallocatechin Gallate), provide antioxidant protection to shield cells from damage. By reducing inflammation, green tea creates a healthier space for cells to repair and grow, while its immune-supporting properties help keep your defenses strong. It also promotes a balanced gut, essential for nutrient absorption and maintaining overall health. This layered support makes green tea a powerful ally in protecting your body's "house."

- **Recommended Amount:** 3 to 4 cups of green tea daily, or 300-400 mg of green tea extract. For those sensitive to caffeine, decaf options are available for both tea and extract, retaining a rich antioxidant content with minimal caffeine.

- **Simple Ways to Include It:** Enjoy hot or iced green tea throughout the day, or try a concentrated green tea extract as a supplement if tea is not a preferred drink.

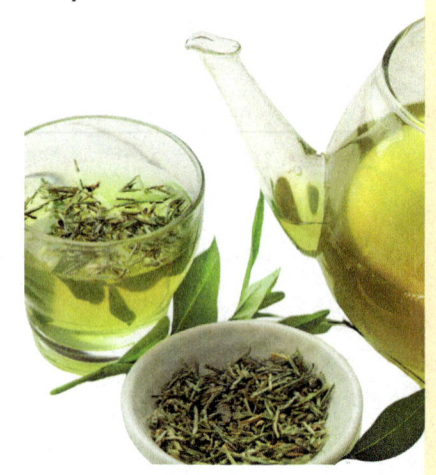

3. Garlic

- **Why It Matters:** Garlic is the all-around handyman, managing repairs, supporting gut health, and boosting immunity while also providing antioxidants. Its sulfur compounds help patch up cellular "cracks," reduce damage from harmful particles, support immune defenses, control inflammation, and nurture good gut bacteria. While leafy greens are strong in detoxifying, garlic's full range equips it to strengthen weak spots throughout the body, reinforcing every part of your "house."

Power Boosters

TOP 5 Nutritional Boosters

Power Boosters

- **Recommended Amount:** 1 to 2 cloves of fresh garlic daily or 600-1,200 mg of garlic extract.
- **Simple Ways to Include It:** Use fresh garlic in cooking, add to dressings or sauces, or try a garlic supplement for added convenience.

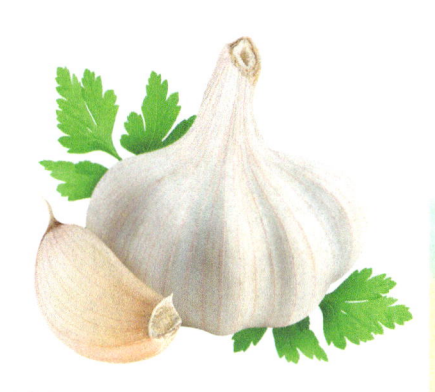

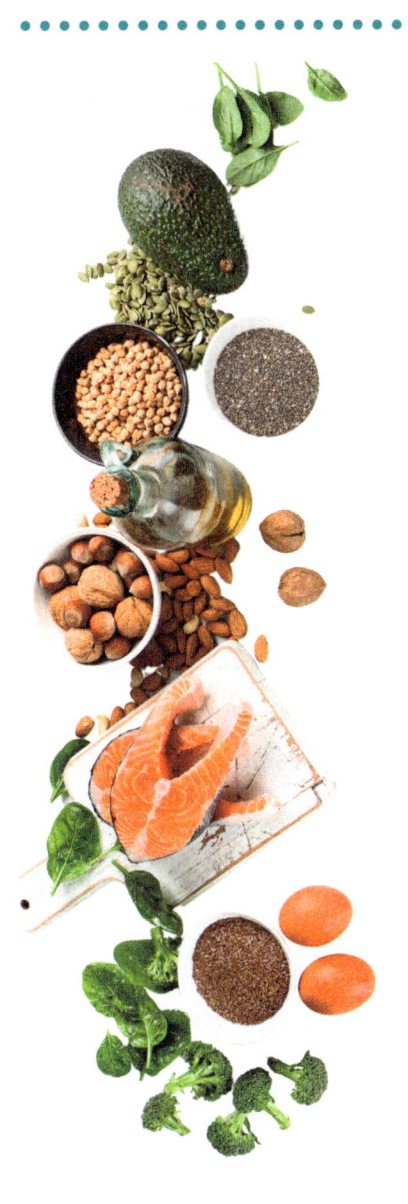

4. Omega-3

- **Why It Matters:** Omega-3s are like structural reinforcements for your house, balancing and stabilizing each part of your body's defenses. These healthy fats protect cells from damage, reduce inflammation, support DNA stability, and enhance immune response. Omega-3s don't just offer general support; they help control harmful cell growth and improve gut health, working across BLOCK to keep your body's foundation strong.
- **Recommended Amount:** 1,000 to 2,000 mg of combined EPA and DHA daily from fish oil or algae oil.
- **Simple Ways to Include It**: Incorporate fatty fish like salmon and sardines into your meals, or take a high-quality fish oil supplement. For a vegan option, try algae oil, which provides EPA and DHA from a plant-based source.

TOP 5 Nutritional Boosters

5. Ginger

- **Why It Matters:** Ginger serves as a caring overseer, helping maintain harmony across all BLOCK pillars. Known for easing inflammation and soothing digestion, ginger also supports immune health, aids in cellular repair, and protects cells from damage. Unlike foods focused on just one job, ginger's diverse qualities strengthen each BLOCK area, promoting a balanced and robust internal environment that keeps your "house" in top shape.

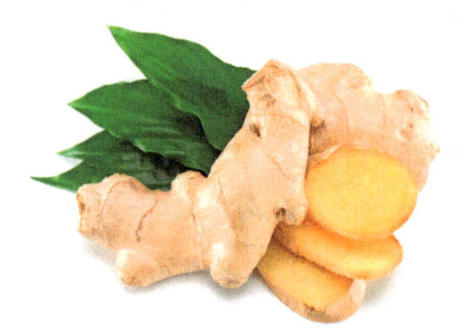

- **Recommended Amount:** 1 to 2 grams of ginger powder daily, or up to 500 mg of ginger extract capsules.
- **Simple Ways to Include It:** Add fresh ginger to tea, smoothies, and stir-fries, or use ginger powder in cooking or baking. Ginger supplements are also available for easy daily intake.

••

These nutritional boosters offer a powerful, concentrated way to strengthen each BLOCK pillar. By incorporating these foods, supplements, or extracts into your routine, you're giving your body extra reinforcements beyond what diet alone provides. To help you integrate these effectively, a detailed dosage guide is available in **Appendix D**, offering safe daily amounts, timing, and forms for each booster. Together with cancer-fighting foods, these boosters help build a strong, resilient foundation, providing added support to each part of your body's "house."

While adding reinforcements is key, it's also vital to avoid foods that weaken the BLOCK pillars. Next, we'll look at the **Top 5 Unhealthy Foods to Limit** and how cutting back can strengthen your body's defenses against cancer.

Power Boosters

TOP 5 Unhealthy Foods to Limit

"When you clear out the clutter in your diet, you make room for the nutrients that truly nourish and protect." – C. Letitia Henry

While healthy foods strengthen your body's defenses, unhealthy ones do the opposite. Imagine a Jenga game where sturdy blocks are replaced with sponges—these weaker pieces may fit but lack stability. Over time, they make the structure wobbly and prone to collapse.

Similarly, too many unhealthy foods can weaken your body's defenses, increasing vulnerability to cancer and other health issues. In this section, we'll explore the top five foods to limit or avoid to protect each BLOCK pillar, making sure your body's "house" remains fortified and strong.

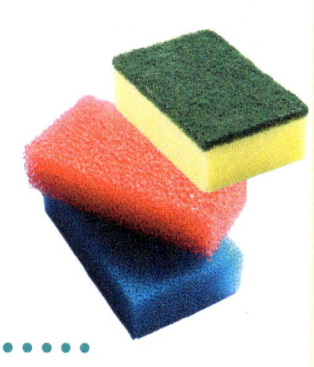

1. Processed Meats

- **Why They're Harmful:** Processed meats like bacon, sausages, hot dogs, and deli meats contain nitrates and nitrites, which can convert into cancer-causing compounds in the body. These foods erode the "paint" or protective layer on your house, allowing harmful elements to penetrate and damage cells.
- **Recommended Limit:** Try to limit processed meats to no more than 1 to 2 servings per month. Frequent consumption is linked to an increased risk of certain cancers, especially colorectal cancer.
- **Healthy Swap:** Choose unprocessed meats that resemble the animal they came from. For example, choose a chicken breast over chicken nuggets, or a whole fish fillet instead of fish sticks. Plant-based protein sources like beans and legumes are also great alternatives.

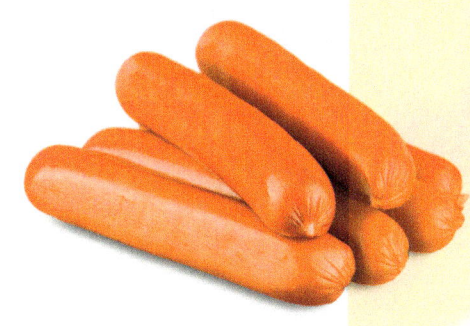

TOP 5 Unhealthy Foods to Limit

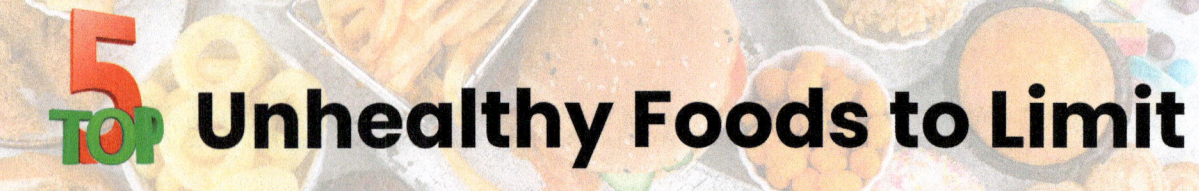

2. Sugary Drinks and Foods

- **Why They're Harmful:** Sugary drinks and foods, such as sodas, candy, and baked goods, can lead to weight gain, inflammation, and insulin resistance, all of which contribute to cancer risk. Consuming these foods is like adding fuel to a fire in your house, causing inflammation to spread, weakening the structure.
- **Recommended Limit:** Women should aim for no more than 25 grams (6 teaspoons) of added sugar daily, and men should limit it to 36 grams (9 teaspoons). For reference, a typical can of soda contains about 39 grams of sugar—more than the recommended daily limit for both men and women.
- **Healthy Swap:** Choose naturally sweetened foods like fresh fruits or yogurt with berries for fiber and nutrients. For beverages, opt for water, herbal teas, or unsweetened drinks to reduce added sugars.

3. Fried Foods

- **Why They're Harmful:** Fried foods, such as French fries, fried chicken, and potato chips, are often cooked at high temperatures, creating harmful compounds like acrylamide. This is like adding weak, cracked pieces to the foundation of your house, compromising its structural integrity and making it harder to repair.
- **Recommended Limit:** Try to limit fried foods to 1-2 servings per week, opting for healthier cooking methods whenever possible. Over time, reducing fried food intake can help protect cells and promote better overall health.
- **Healthy Swap:** Choose baked, roasted, or air-fried versions that provide the crunch or texture you enjoy without the health risks associated with frying.

TOP 5 Unhealthy Foods to Limit

4. Alcohol

- **Why It's Harmful:** Alcohol is a known carcinogen, damaging DNA and impairing the body's ability to repair itself. It's like sabotaging the house's security system, allowing harmful "intruders" in and making it difficult for the immune system to control unhealthy cell changes.
- **Recommended Limit:** Women should limit alcohol to no more than one drink per day, and men to no more than two drinks per day. Reducing or avoiding alcohol altogether can significantly lower cancer risk.
- **Healthy Swap:** Choose Concord grape juice, which offers beneficial antioxidants similar to those in red wine, without the alcohol. Other satisfying, alcohol-free alternatives include sparkling water, herbal teas, non-alcoholic beers, and mocktails made with fresh fruits and herbs.

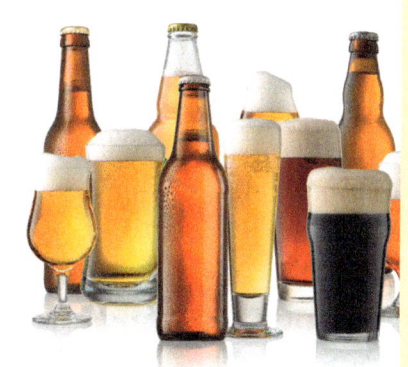

5. Red Meat

- **Why It's Harmful:** High intake of red meat (like beef, pork, and lamb) has been associated with an increased risk of colorectal and other cancers, partly due to compounds formed during cooking and high levels of saturated fat. This saturated fat can clog the body's "plumbing" system, making it difficult to flush out toxins and adding to inflammation over time.
- **Recommended Limit:** Consume no more than 500 grams (about 1 pound) of cooked red meat per week—roughly one 5-ounce serving, three times a week.

TOP 5 Unhealthy Foods to Limit

- **Healthy Swap:** Opt for lean protein sources like skinless poultry (chicken, turkey, Cornish hen), fish (salmon, tuna, or cod), or plant-based proteins like beans and lentils for a balanced, heart-healthy option.

    If choosing red meat, go for leaner cuts such as sirloin, tenderloin, or round for beef; tenderloin or loin chops for pork; and loin or leg cuts for lamb. Goat meat is also a naturally leaner red meat alternative.

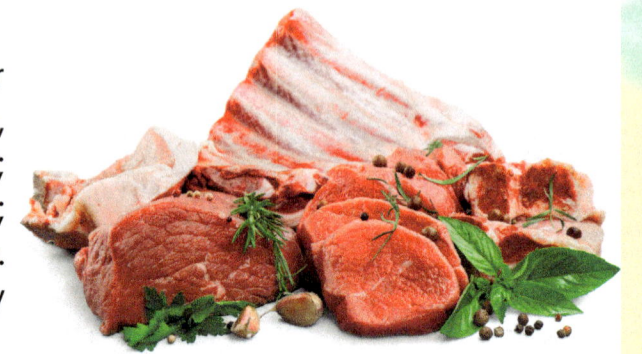

• •

By limiting or avoiding these unhealthy foods, you're removing weak "blocks" from your body's foundation, ensuring that each part of the BLOCK structure remains strong. Small changes, like opting for whole foods and minimizing processed or fried options, can make a meaningful difference. Every choice you make helps reinforce the structure, just as replacing sponges with solid pieces would stabilize a Jenga tower. For practical ideas on healthier choices, see **Appendix E** for a guide to simple swaps that support each BLOCK pillar.

Building a strong, cancer-resistant foundation goes beyond diet alone. In the next section, we'll explore the **Top 5 Cancer-Fighting Habits** that work in tandem with nutritious foods to further reinforce each BLOCK pillar. From stress management to regular exercise, these habits create an environment where your body can thrive.

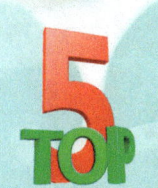

TOP 5 Cancer-Fighting Habits

"Small, consistent habits are the daily bricks that fortify the foundation of lifelong health." – C. Letitia Henry

In addition to a balanced diet, certain lifestyle habits help strengthen the BLOCK pillars that keep your body resilient and help you fight against cancer naturally. These habits act like daily maintenance, just as regular upkeep keeps a house strong over time. Simple, consistent practices—such as staying hydrated, managing stress, getting enough sleep, exercising, and avoiding smoking—support each pillar in unique ways, with some overlapping benefits.

In this section, we'll connect each habit with a specific BLOCK pillar, although many offer benefits across multiple areas, providing a strong, everyday defense for your health.

1. Stay Hydrated

- **Why It Matters:** Water acts as the "sealant" that protects your house from the wear and tear of daily life, helping antioxidants flow through your body to protect cells. Free radicals, like harsh weather elements—sun, rain, or wind—wear down the protective paint on your house (your body), leaving it vulnerable to damage. Staying hydrated enables antioxidants to work effectively, keeping your cells protected. Hydration also ensures nutrients are properly absorbed and delivered where needed, helping to "seal in" your body's defenses and prevent structural damage from within.

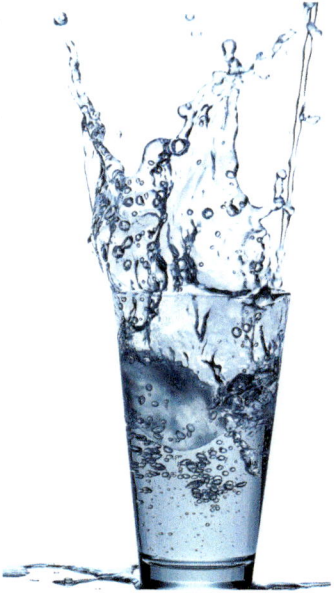

Healthy Lifestyle Habits

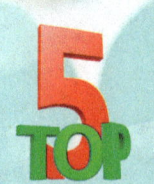

TOP 5 Cancer-Fighting Habits

- **How Much and When:** Aim for about 8-10 cups (64-80 ounces) of water daily, though individual needs may vary based on activity level, climate, and overall health. Start your day with a glass of water to rehydrate after sleep, then spread your intake evenly throughout the day. Drinking water with meals and between activities helps maintain hydration consistently.

2. Manage Stress

- **Why It Matters:** Stress acts like a spark that can start an inflammation "fire" inside your body, which, if left unchecked, can cause lasting damage. When stress is prolonged, the "fire" continues to burn, weakening your cells and making them more susceptible to harm. Managing stress is like having a built-in fire extinguisher to keep these flames low, protecting your body's healthy cells and minimizing potential damage. By keeping inflammation under control, you prevent it from spreading and creating an environment that supports cancer cell growth.
- **How Much and When:** Dedicate at least 10-15 minutes daily to stress-relieving activities, such as meditation, deep breathing, journaling, or light physical activity like walking. Start or end your day with a calming routine, like journaling or breathing exercises, and practice shorter techniques—such as a few deep breaths—whenever stressful situations arise throughout the day.

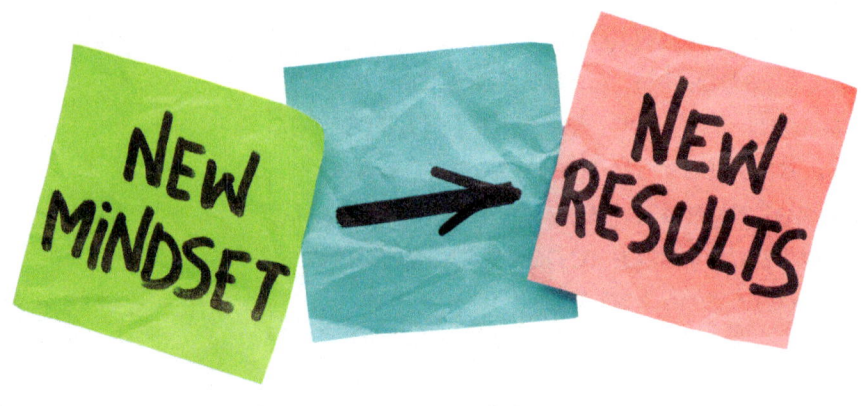

Healthy Lifestyle Habits

TOP 5 Cancer-Fighting Habits

3. Get Enough Sleep

- **Why It Matters:** Sleep is your body's "repair time," like when cracks in the house's foundation are patched up to keep the structure strong. During sleep, your body fixes cell damage and repairs DNA, preventing small issues from growing into larger structural problems. Just like regular maintenance keeps a home's foundation solid, quality sleep strengthens your immune system and repairs cells, reducing the risk of mutations and making sure your body can respond to health challenges.
- **How Much and When:** Adults should aim for 7–9 hours of sleep each night for optimal health benefits. Maintain a consistent sleep schedule by going to bed and waking up at the same times daily, even on weekends. Establish a relaxing nighttime routine to help your body wind down, signaling that it's time for rest.

4. Exercise Regularly

- **Why It Matters:** Exercise is like regularly testing your house's security system, ensuring it's active and responsive. Physical activity strengthens the immune "security system" that monitors cell growth and eliminates abnormal cells before they cause issues. Regular exercise lowers cancer risk by helping your body identify and eliminate harmful cells quickly, keeping everything under control just as a security system would keep intruders out of a well-protected home.
- **How Much and When:** Aim for at least 150 minutes of moderate-intensity exercise (like brisk walking) or 75 minutes of vigorous-intensity exercise (like jogging) each week, along with two days of muscle-strengthening activities. To achieve this, consider daily 20–30 minute sessions, with rest days as needed to allow for recovery.

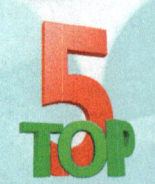

TOP 5 Cancer-Fighting Habits

5. Avoid Smoking

- **Why It Matters:** Smoking introduces toxins that clog your body's "plumbing," much like debris buildup in pipes that can eventually cause a backup. These toxins make it harder for your body to remove waste, allowing damaging compounds to accumulate, which can lead to serious problems, including cancer. Avoiding smoking allows your body's "plumbing" to stay clear, keeping your system clean and functioning optimally.
- **How Much and When:** Complete cessation is the goal, as even minimal smoking or secondhand smoke exposure can increase cancer risk. Other types of smoking to avoid include vaping, hookah, e-cigarettes, marijuana smoking, and heated tobacco products (HTPs), each of which introduces harmful chemicals that may increase cancer risk. Avoiding these whenever possible supports a healthier lifestyle, and resources or support groups can provide assistance with quitting.

•••••••••••••••••••••••••••••••••••••

Incorporating these cancer-fighting lifestyle habits is like routine maintenance on your house, helping to keep every part of the structure solid and reliable. Small, consistent actions strengthen the BLOCK pillars, supporting overall wellness and lowering cancer risk. For quick reference, check **Appendices F, G, H, I, and J**, where you'll find resources on hydration, stress relief, sleep hygiene, exercise, and quit-smoking support.

Understanding factors that influence cancer risk is essential. In the next section, we'll explore the **Top 5 Cancer Risk Factors**, including sun exposure, health screenings, and environmental awareness—empowering you to make effective choices for lasting health.

TOP 5 Cancer Risk Factors

"Awareness is the first step in prevention—understanding risks empowers us to protect our health." – C. Letitia Henry

Understanding and managing key cancer risk factors can make a significant difference in your health. This section covers five crucial areas—genetic awareness, weight management, health screenings, environmental awareness, and sun exposure. By focusing on each of these factors, you can take steps to reduce your cancer risk.

1. Genetic Awareness

- **Why It Matters:** Genetics can play a substantial role in cancer risk. While you can't change your genes, knowing your family history allows you to tailor preventive strategies. Certain genetic tests, like BRCA1 and BRCA2 for breast and ovarian cancer risk, offer insights into inherited gene mutations that may elevate cancer risk. A study from the National Cancer Institute in 2009 found that people with BRCA mutations who took preventive steps lowered their cancer risk by as much as 90%.

- **How to Approach It:** Start by gathering information about your family's medical history. If you have relatives who developed cancer, consider discussing genetic testing with a healthcare provider. With personalized guidance, you'll have a better sense of which screenings or lifestyle adjustments are most beneficial for you.

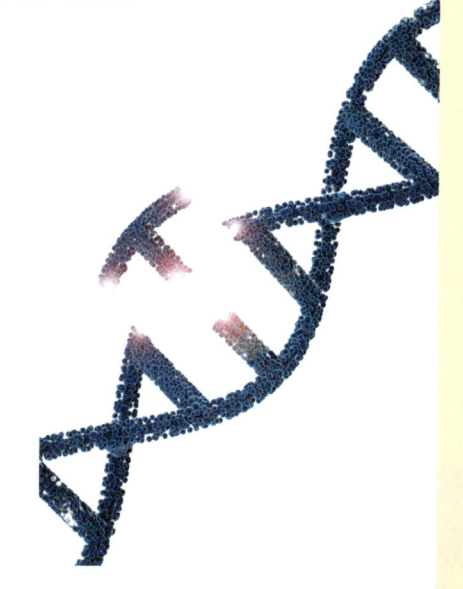

Risk Awareness

TOP 5 Cancer Risk Factors

2. Weight Management Awareness

- **Why It Matters:** Excessive weight can increase cancer risk, particularly for cancers like breast, colon, and liver. Studies show that maintaining a healthy weight reduces cancer risk, while obesity can lead to chronic inflammation, an environment that may encourage cancer cell growth. Body Mass Index (BMI) is a common indicator; a BMI over 30 is generally considered obese, signaling increased cancer risk.

- **How to Assess It:** Calculate your BMI or ask a healthcare provider for a comprehensive evaluation. If your BMI indicates an elevated risk, consider reaching out for professional support to create a weight management plan. Managing weight helps keep your body balanced and reduces strain on organs, contributing to overall wellness.

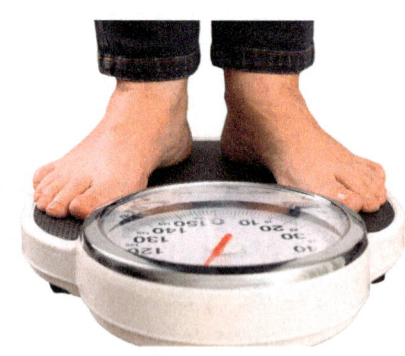

3. Regular Health Screenings

- **Why They Matter:** Health screenings are essential for early cancer detection. Studies have shown that routine screenings can significantly reduce cancer death rates; for example, regular colonoscopies reduce the risk of dying from colorectal cancer by up to 68%. Screenings help catch cancer in its earliest stages, improving the effectiveness of treatment and chances of recovery.

- **Screening Recommendations:** Common screenings include mammograms, colonoscopies, and skin checks, with frequency based on age, family history, and risk level. Consult your healthcare provider for a personalized screening schedule, and aim to stay consistent. Regular screenings offer peace of mind and enable early intervention if needed.

TOP 5 Cancer Risk Factors

4. Environmental Awareness

- **Why It Matters:** Daily exposure to environmental factors like pesticides, chemicals, and pollution can increase cancer risk. Studies have shown that reducing exposure to certain industrial chemicals can lead to lower cancer rates. For instance, research found that factory workers who were frequently exposed to benzene—a chemical used in manufacturing plastics, detergents, and other everyday products—had a higher risk of developing leukemia. When steps were taken to limit exposure, including improved ventilation, protective gear, and stricter safety regulations, the cancer rates in these workers significantly declined.
- **Practical Tips:** Choose organic produce when possible to reduce pesticide exposure, ventilate indoor spaces to lessen indoor air pollution, add an air-purifying plant to promote cleaner indoor air, and filter your drinking water. Making small adjustments can significantly reduce harmful environmental exposures and help your body stay well-protected.

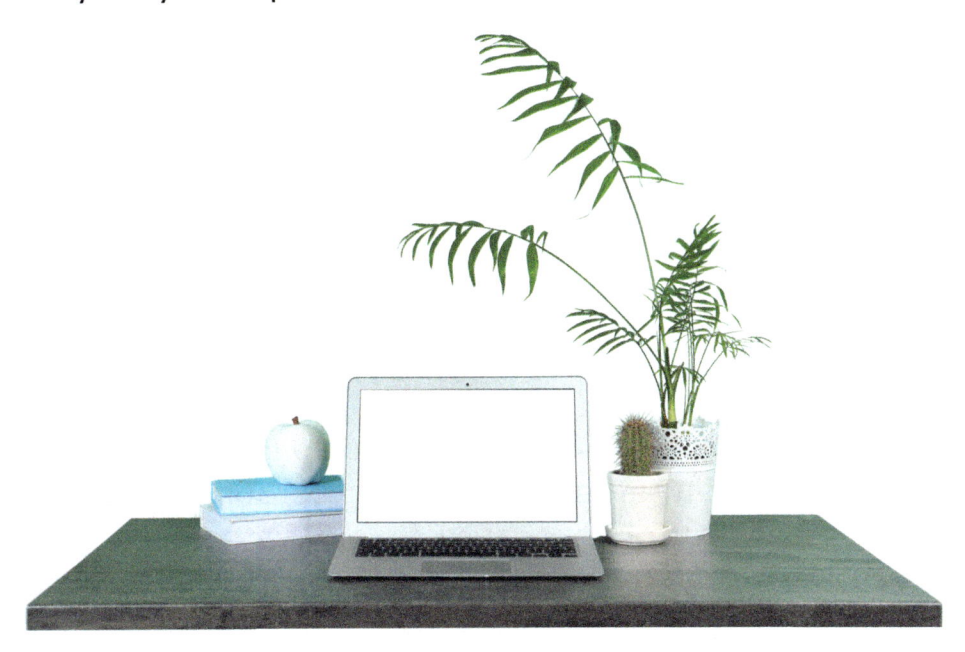

Top 5 Cancer Risk Factors

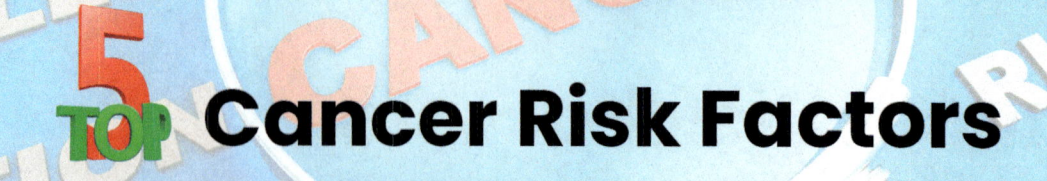

5. Sun Exposure Awareness

- **Why It Matters:** Sunlight is a natural source of vitamin D, essential for immune function and overall health. However, prolonged exposure raises the risk of skin cancer. The American Cancer Society recommends short sun exposure between 10 a.m. and 2 p.m. for optimal vitamin D production, but this is also when UV rays are strongest. To safely get sunlight during these hours, wear protective clothing like long sleeves, hats, and sunglasses to shield your skin from excessive exposure. It's also a myth that darker skin is immune to damage; all skin types benefit from sun protection.
- **Sun Safety Tips:** To maintain balanced vitamin D levels, aim for 10-15 minutes of sun exposure daily. If you are outside longer, apply sunscreen with at least SPF 30 or wear protective clothing. Regularly using these protective measures supports skin health for everyone.
- **Sun Safety Tips:** To maintain balanced vitamin D levels, aim for 10-15 minutes of sun exposure daily. If you are outside longer, apply sunscreen with at least SPF 30 or wear protective clothing. Regularly using these protective measures supports skin health for everyone.

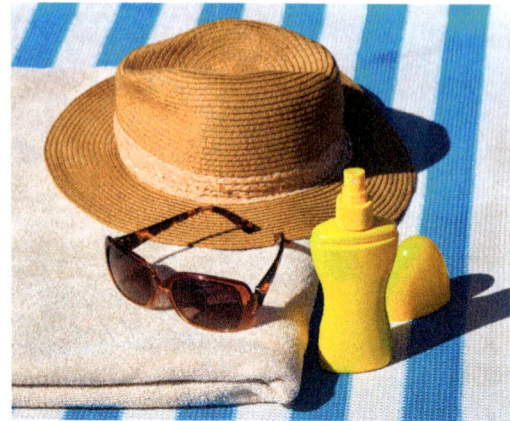

Addressing these risk factors proactively can help lower your cancer risk. Small changes—whether scheduling a screening, checking weight indicators, or reducing exposure to environmental toxins—empower you to make healthier choices that align with long-term wellness.

Conclusion

Recap of BLOCK Pillars

Each of the BLOCK pillars represents a key aspect of a fortified, cancer-preventive lifestyle. The five core practices we just discussed help keep these pillars strong, helping create a solid base for your overall health. Let's briefly revisit each pillar to see how they collectively protect you.

BLOCK Recap

B - Boost Barrier: Foods and nutrients rich in antioxidants act as a protective coating on your cells, shielding them from harmful free radicals that wear down your body over time.

L - Lessen the Damage: Anti-inflammatory choices help keep "fires" in check, calming inflammation so it doesn't harm healthy cells or create an environment where cancer cells can thrive.

O - Oversee Repairs: Nutrients and lifestyle habits that support DNA repair ensure that small "cracks" or cellular damage are swiftly patched up, keeping your body's foundation strong.

C - Control Growth: Exercise, immune-boosting foods, and healthy habits regulate cell growth, helping your immune system stay vigilant and removing abnormal cells before they pose a risk.

K - Keep It Clean: A balanced diet, fiber, and hydration help maintain a clean and efficient "plumbing system" within your body, removing toxins and reducing cancer risk.

Together, these pillars form a sturdy foundation, much like the strong walls of a well-built house, reinforcing your body's natural defenses against cancer.

Putting BLOCK into Pratice

Call to Action

Now that you understand the BLOCK pillars, let's turn this knowledge into action. Refer to your BLOCK Self-Check results to help you decide which small steps to take. If your Self-Check showed a low score in any area, start by adding one food, habit, or booster from that category—like leafy greens in meals, a new exercise, or daily stress relief. Each small, consistent change strengthens your body, building a foundation for lasting health.

Remember the Jenga game analogy we used: each piece you place carefully strengthens your house (your body). By focusing on solid, cancer-fighting foods and habits, you're creating a structure that is better equipped to withstand life's wear and tear. However, just as in the Jenga game, there are moments when unexpected challenges come along. Sometimes, even with every solid piece in place, an outside force—like a hard bump to the table—can cause the pieces to fall. This is a reminder that while we can reduce our cancer risk through intentional choices, some factors remain beyond our control. However, the stronger the foundation, the better the stability and chance to weather the storm.

Let the BLOCK pillars guide you as a daily reminder to build a life that prioritizes prevention, balance, and resilience. By committing to these small, meaningful steps, you're actively investing in a healthier future. Remember, your health is your greatest asset, and every action you take strengthens the foundation that supports it. Take the first step today, and know that each piece you add brings you closer to a life of lasting wellness. For a daily routine that incorporates cancer-fighting foods, nutritional boosters, hydration, stress relief, and more, see **Appendix K: BLOCK Pillar Plan** for inspiration.

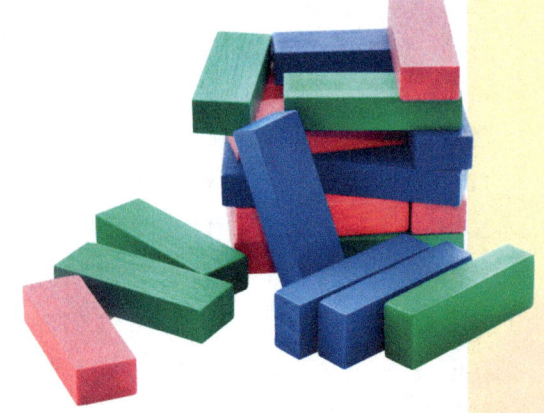

Building a Support Team

"True wellness is a journey built step-by-step, with guidance and care turning goals into lasting foundations." – C. Letitia Henry

As you start incorporating the BLOCK pillars into your daily life, remember that support is available. Consulting with a health professional—such as a dietitian, exercise physiologist, life coach, therapist, or preventive care specialist—can provide you with personalized guidance to help you make choices that fit your lifestyle and address any challenges along the way. Working with a professional can offer reassurance, strengthen your approach, and help you focus on what truly matters: your well-being and future. For added support, see **Appendix L: Cancer Resources** for trusted organizations and tools to assist your journey.

As you move forward, remember that each choice you make strengthens your health journey. May every step guided by the BLOCK pillars bring you closer to a life of lasting wellness, balance, and vitality. Wishing you all the best on this path to a fulfilling, vibrant future centered on health and happiness.

Appendices: What's Inside

Appendix A – BLOCK Self-Check...39

Appendix B – BLOCK Shopping List & Recipes..........45

Appendix C – Cancer Nutrition Myths..........................50

Appendix D – Nutrition Boosters Guide.......................53

Appendix E – Healthy Swap Guide................................59

Appendix F – Hydration Essentials...............................62

Appendix G – Stress-Relief Practices...........................66

Appendix H – Sleep Hygiene Tips.................................68

Appendix I – Weekly Exercise Guide............................69

Appendix J – Quit Smoking Support.............................71

Appendix K – BLOCK Pillar Plan....................................72

Appendix L – Cancer Resources....................................74

Appendix A

BLOCK Self-Check

This self-assessment helps you reflect on your habits across key lifestyle areas, including healthy foods, nutritional boosters, limiting unhealthy foods, beneficial habits, and awareness of cancer risk factors.

Instructions:
Consider your habits over the past month to get a realistic view of your current lifestyle. For each question, choose the response that best describes your recent habits, selecting only one answer per question. At the end, use the scoring guide to calculate your total score, which will help you identify areas for growth and guide your journey toward improved health and reduced cancer risk.

1. How often do you eat leafy greens like spinach, kale, or Swiss chard?
   A. Rarely or never
   B. Occasionally (1-2 times per week)
   C. Regularly (3-4 times per week)
   D. Consistently (daily)

2. How often do you include cruciferous vegetables (like broccoli, cauliflower, or Brussels sprouts) in your meals?
   A. Rarely or never
   B. Occasionally (1-2 times per week)
   C. Regularly (3-4 times per week)
   D. Consistently (daily)

3. How often do you eat berries (like blueberries, strawberries, or raspberries)?
   A. Rarely or never
   B. Occasionally (1-2 times per week)
   C. Regularly (3-4 times per week)
   D. Consistently (daily)

4. Do you include beans or legumes (like lentils, chickpeas, or black beans) in your meals?
   A. Rarely or never
   B. Occasionally (1-2 times per week)
   C. Regularly (3-4 times per week)
   D. Consistently (daily)

5. How often do you consume nuts or seeds (like walnuts, chia seeds, or flaxseeds)?
   A. Rarely or never
   B. Occasionally (1-2 times per week)
   C. Regularly (3-4 times per week)
   D. Consistently (daily)

6. How often do you consume foods high in omega-3s, like salmon, chia seeds, or walnuts?
   A. Rarely or never
   B. Occasionally (1-2 times per week)
   C. Regularly (3-4 times per week)
   D. Consistently (daily)

7. Do you consume green tea or take green tea extract regularly?
   A. Rarely or never
   B. Occasionally (1-2 times per week)
   C. Regularly (3-4 times per week)
   D. Consistently (daily)

8. How often do you include turmeric in your meals or take it as a supplement?
   A. Rarely or never
   B. Occasionally (1-2 times per week)
   C. Regularly (3-4 times per week)
   D. Consistently (daily)

9. How often do you include garlic in your meals or take it as a supplement?
   A. Rarely or never
   B. Occasionally (1-2 times per week)
   C. Regularly (3-4 times per week)
   D. Consistently (daily)

10. How often do you consume ginger (either fresh, powdered, or as a supplement)?
   A. Rarely or never
   B. Occasionally (1-2 times per week)
   C. Regularly (3-4 times per week)
   D. Consistently (daily)

11. How often do you eat processed meats (like hot dogs, bacon, or deli meats)?
   A. Consistently (daily)
   B. Regularly (3-4 times a week)
   C. Occasionally (1-2 times a week)
   D. Rarely or never

12. How often do you consume sugary drinks (like soda, sweetened teas, or energy drinks)?
   A. Consistently (daily)
   B. Regularly (3-4 times a week)
   C. Occasionally (1-2 times a week)
   D. Rarely or never

13. How often do you eat fried foods?
   A. Consistently (daily)
   B. Regularly (3-4 times a week)
   C. Occasionally (1-2 times a week)
   D. Rarely or never

14. How often do you consume high-sugar desserts (like pastries, cookies, or ice cream)?
   A. Consistently (daily)
   B. Regularly (3-4 times a week)
   C. Occasionally (1-2 times a week)
   D. Rarely or never

15. How often do you eat refined grains (like white bread, pasta, or rice)?
   A. Consistently (daily)
   B. Regularly (3-4 times a week)
   C. Occasionally (1-2 times a week)
   D. Rarely or never

16. How many days per week do you engage in moderate physical activity, like brisk walking or biking?
    A. Rarely or never
    B. Occasionally (1-2 days per week)
    C. Regularly (3-4 days per week)
    D. Consistently (5 or more days per week)

17. How often do you practice stress-relief techniques, such as meditation or deep breathing?
    A. Rarely or never
    B. Occasionally (1-2 times per week)
    C. Regularly (3-4 times per week)
    D. Consistently (daily)

18. How many hours of sleep do you typically get each night?
    A. Fewer than 5 hours
    B. 10+ hours
    C. 5-6 hours
    D. 7-9 hours

19. How often do you consume at least 8 glasses of water daily?
    A. Rarely or never
    B. Occasionally (1-2 times per week)
    C. Regularly (3-4 times per week)
    D. Consistently (daily)

20. How would you describe your smoking or secondhand smoke exposure?
    A. Frequently
    B. Occasionally
    C. Rarely
    D. Never

21. How often do you follow through with recommended cancer screenings (e.g., mammograms, colonoscopies) for your age and risk level?
    A. Rarely or never
    B. Occasionally (when it comes up)
    C. Regularly (on a recommended schedule)
    D. Consistently (stay on track with all screening schedules)

22. Are you aware of your family's cancer history, and have you considered genetic testing if there's a high risk?
    A. I haven't explored this area yet
    B. I know some family history but haven't looked into genetic testing
    C. I am aware of family risks but haven't tested
    D. I know my family history well and have considered or done genetic testing

23. How often do you try to reduce your exposure to potential carcinogens like pesticides, industrial chemicals, or air pollutants?
    A. Rarely or never
    B. Sometimes, but it's not a priority
    C. Often, I am somewhat mindful of limiting exposure
    D. Consistently, I actively work to limit my exposure

24. Are you aware of how your weight impacts cancer risk, and do you monitor your weight regularly?
    A. I don't monitor or consider my weight for cancer prevention
    B. I'm somewhat aware but rarely check my weight
    C. I am aware and sometimes monitor my weight
    D. I actively manage my weight and track it regularly

25. Do you take steps to protect your skin from excessive sun exposure (like wearing sunscreen or protective clothing)?
    A. Rarely or never
    B. Occasionally, but it's not consistent
    C. I'm mindful of sun exposure and try to protect myself
    D. Consistently, I always use sun protection

Cancer Prevention Score

Scoring System

For each question, assign points as follows:
A = 0 points
B = 1 point
C = 2 points
D = 3 points

Total Points Available: 75 points

Use the following scale to interpret your score and identify areas for improvement:

- **60–75 points – Solid Foundation:** You're taking comprehensive steps to lower cancer risk. Continue these habits to maintain a strong foundation for health.
- **45–59 points – Stable Structure:** You're aware of many risk factors and implementing effective practices. Focus on areas with lower scores to boost your efforts.
- **30–44 points – Needs Strengthening:** You have some good practices but could benefit from addressing more areas consistently. Try to build habits that will strengthen your cancer-preventive lifestyle.
- **Below 30 points – At-Risk Foundation:** Identify specific areas to improve and consider small, manageable changes. Each step you take can make a positive difference in reducing cancer risk.

Your score provides a snapshot of your current health habits. If you scored lower in some areas, start with small, simple changes to build lasting benefits. If you scored well, keep reinforcing those positive habits. Each step moves you closer to lifelong wellness. As you read the book, you'll discover how each food, habit, and lifestyle choice you explored in the questionnaire can help reduce your cancer risk and support your health journey.

Appendix B

BLOCK Shopping List & Recipes

This appendix provides a complete, categorized shopping list and a selection of nutrient-dense recipes to support your BLOCK pillars. Use this guide as a quick reference to stock your kitchen and prepare meals that reinforce your body's natural defenses.

What's Inside

Comprehensive Shopping List: Organized by food group, each category includes essential ingredients rich in nutrients aligned with the BLOCK pillars.

Cancer-Preventive Recipes: Easy-to-follow recipes that integrate top cancer-fighting ingredients, making it simple to add protective foods to your daily meals.

Practical Tips

Use the shopping list to streamline your grocery trips, focusing on ingredients that support your health goals. Then, try out the recipes to enjoy meals packed with nutrients that benefit each BLOCK area.

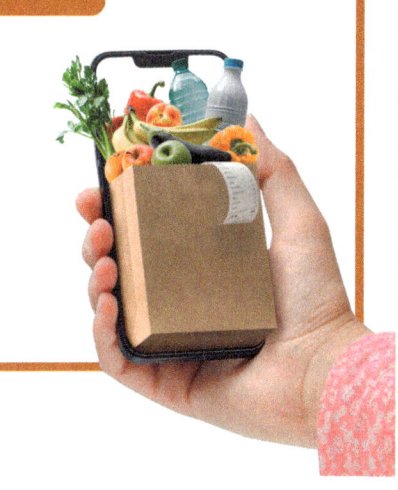

BLOCK Shopping List

Vegetables

Cruciferous Vegetables:
Bok choy
Broccoli
Brussels sprouts
Cabbage
Cauliflower
Radishes
Watercress

Leafy Greens:
Amaranth (kallaloo)
Arugula
Collard greens
Kale
Lettuce (romaine)
Mustard greens
Spinach
Swiss chard
Turnip greens

Other Vegetables:
Bell peppers
Breadfruit
Carrots
Cassava (yuca)
Plantain
Sweet potatoes
Tomatoes
Yams
Zucchini

Fruits

Berries:
Acerola cherries
Blackberries
Blueberries
Cranberries
Guavaberries
Raspberries
Strawberries

Other Fruits:
Apples
Bananas
Citrus fruits
Guavas
Mangos
Papayas
Pears
Pineapples
Pomegranates
Soursops
Tamarinds

Whole Grains

Barley
Brown rice
Bulgur
Farro
Oats
Quinoa
Whole wheat

Beans & Peas

Black beans
Black-eyed peas
Chickpeas
Lima beans
Lentils
Mung beans
Navy beans
Pigeon peas
Red kidney beans

Nuts & Seeds

Almonds
Brazil nuts
Cashews
Chia seeds
Flaxseeds
Pecans
Pumpkin seeds
Sunflower seeds
Walnuts

Fats & Oils

Avocado
Avocado oil
Flaxseed oil
Oil spray
Olive oil (extra-virgin)
Sesame oil

Fatty Fish

Herring
Mackerel
Salmon
Sardines
Trout
Tuna

Probiotics

Yogurt
Kefir
Sauerkraut
Kimchi

Prebiotics

Garlic (see Herbs)
Onions
Leeks

Herbs & Spices

Cayenne pepper
Cinnamon
Garlic
Ginger
Green tea leaves or bags
Rosemary
Thyme
Turmeric

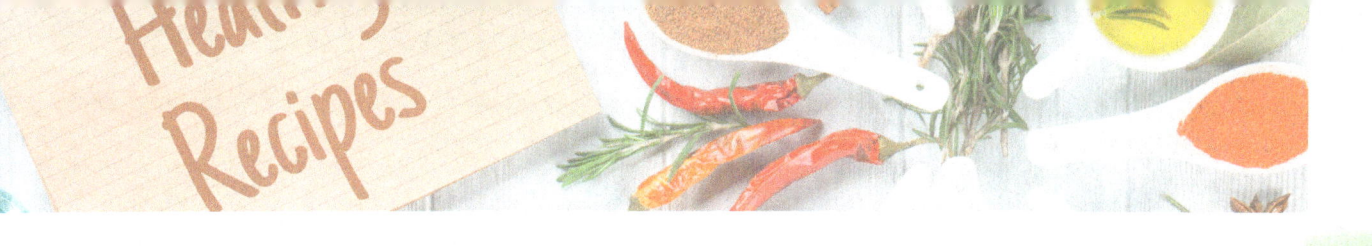

Mango-Banana Oat Bars

Prep Time: 15 minutes   Total Time: 40 minutes   Yield: 10 servings

Ingredients

- 2 small bananas, ripe
- 1/2 cup almond butter or other nut/seed butter
- 2 eggs
- 1 tsp vanilla extract
- 2 Tbsp coconut oil, melted
- 3 Tbsp honey
- 1 1/2 cups oats, quick-cook
- 1/2 cup almond flour
- 1/2 cup coconut flour
- 1/4 cup flax meal
- 1/2 tsp baking powder
- 1/2 tsp baking soda
- 1/3 cup dried mango, diced
- 1/2 cup dark chocolate or cacao nibs

Instructions

Prep
1. Preheat oven to 350°F and line a baking sheet with parchment paper.
2. Peel and chop the bananas
3. Dice the dried mango.

Make
1. In a blender or food processor, combine the bananas, almond butter, eggs, vanilla extract, coconut oil, and honey. Blend until smooth.
2. In a large mixing bowl, whisk together oats, flours, flax meal, baking powder, baking soda, and mango.
3. Create a well in the center of the dry ingredients and pour in the banana mixture. Stir until just combined, then fold in the chocolate or cacao nibs.
4. Scoop 1/4 cup of batter onto the prepared baking sheet, shaping each scoop into bars.
5. Bake for 15-18 minutes or until edges are golden brown.
6. Cool on a wire rack.

Pumpkin Spice Nutty Muesli

Prep Time: 10 minutes   Total Time: 10 minutes   Yield: 8 servings

Ingredients

- 1/4 cup pecans, chopped
- 1/4 cup walnuts, chopped
- 4 dates, pitted and chopped
- 2 cups oats, rolled
- 2 Tbsp chia seeds
- 1/4 cup pumpkin seeds, raw
- 1/4 cup dried papaya, finely chopped
- 1 tsp pumpkin spice, ground
- 1/4 tsp cinnamon, ground
- 1/4 tsp allspice
- Salt, to taste

Instructions

Prep
1. Chop pecans and walnuts
2. Chop dates and dried papaya.

Make
1. Add all ingredients to a large bowl and stir together. Store in an airtight container until ready to eat.
2. Try these serving options:
   - Overnight Oats: Soak the muesli in milk of your choice overnight.
   - Morning Cereal: Serve with milk of your choice, adding fresh fruit if desired.

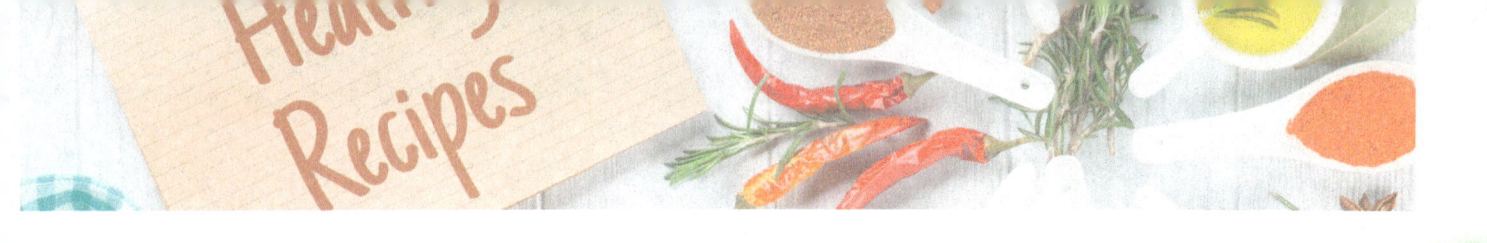

Cinnamon Nut Spice Granola

Prep Time: 5 minutes Total Time: 10 minutes Yield: 6 servings

Ingredients

- 1 cup walnuts, raw, chopped
- 12 Medjool dates, pitted and chopped
- 1 cup oats, rolled
- 1/4 cup coconut flakes, unsweetened
- 1 Tbsp sunflower seeds
- 1 tsp vanilla extract or mixed essence
- 1/2 tsp cinnamon, ground
- Salt, to taste

Instructions

Prep

1. Pit and chop dates.

Make

1. Add walnuts to the food processor and pulse until roughly chopped.
2. Add dates and pulse until combined with walnuts.
3. Add the remaining ingredients and pulse until well combined.
4. Add a few pinches of salt, if desired.
5. Pour mixture onto a baking sheet and separate with fingers. Let air dry for about four hours.
6. Place in an airtight container and store in the refrigerator for up to two weeks.

Spinach and Lima Beans

Prep Time: 10 minutes Total Time: 15 minutes Yield: 4 servings

Ingredients

- 8 cup spinach, chopped
- 1/4 cup sweet onion, chopped
- 4 cloves garlic, minced or pressed
- 1 Tbsp fresh thyme, chopped
- 1 Tbsp Caribbean green seasoning (optional)
- 1/4 tsp scotch bonnet pepper, seeded and finely chopped
- 1 1/2 cups lima beans, canned, drained and rinsed
- 2 Tbsp olive oil
- 2 cup vegetable broth
- Salt, to taste
- Black pepper, to taste
- 2 Tbsp pine nuts

Instructions

Prep

1. Chop spinach, onion, thyme, and scotch bonnet pepper.
2. Mince garlic.
3. Drain and rinse lima beans.

Make

1. Heat olive oil in a large sauté pan over medium heat. Sauté onion until soft and fragrant, about 2 minutes. Stir in garlic, thyme, green seasoning, and scotch bonnet pepper; sauté until aromatic.
2. Add spinach and cook until wilted, about 1 minute.
3. Stir in lima beans and vegetable broth. Let simmer until the liquid reduces by half and the spinach is tender, about 5 minutes.
4. Season with salt and black pepper to taste.
5. Serve with pine nuts.

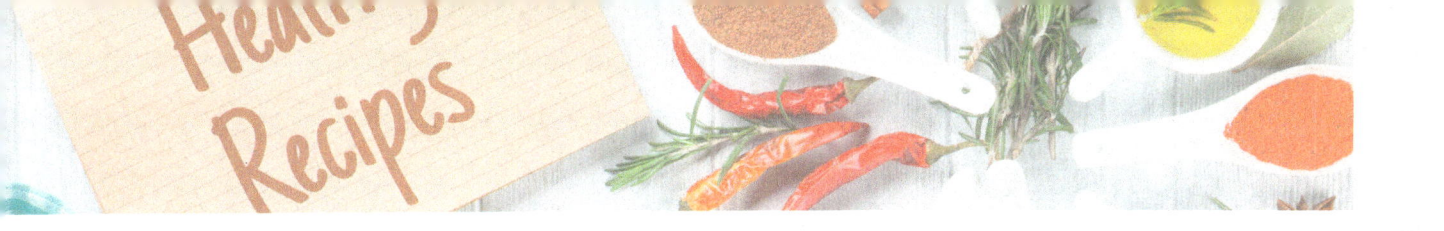

Seed Crusted Salmon with Lentils & Greens

Prep Time: 15 minutes   Total Time: 30 minutes   Yield: 4 servings

Lentils and Greens

Ingredients

- 2 Tbsp olive oil
- 2 cloves garlic, minced
- 2 carrots, peeled and chopped
- 1 1/2 cups canned lentils, drained and rinsed
- 1 lemon, juiced
- 1/2 tsp turmeric
- 1/2 tsp fresh thyme, chopped
- 8 cups kale (or amaranth), spines removed and torn into bite-sized pieces
- 2 scallions, chopped
- Salt and black pepper, to taste

Instructions

Prep

1. Mince garlic and chop thyme leaves and scallions.
2. Peel and chop carrots.
3. Juice lemon.
4. Wash kale or amaranth, remove spines, and tear it into bite-sized pieces.

Make

1. In a large sauté pan, heat olive oil over medium heat and sauté garlic until fragrant.
2. Add carrots, lentils, lemon juice, turmeric, thyme, and amaranth (if using). Stir and continue to sauté over low heat until carrots are tender and amaranth begins to soften.
3. If using kale, add it along with the scallions at this point. Stir to combine, then cover the pan with a lid. Let stand until the greens wilt, approximately 5 more minutes.
4. For softer greens, cook on low for an additional few minutes.
5. Season with salt and pepper to taste, and serve immediately.

Salmon

Ingredients

- 2 lb salmon, filets, cut into portions
- 1 Tbsp olive oil
- 1 Tbsp all-purpose Caribbean blend
- Salt, to taste
- Black pepper, to taste
- 2 Tbsp pumpkin seeds, finely chopped
- 2 Tbsp sesame seeds

Instructions

Prep

1. Preheat oven to 350° F and line a baking sheet with parchment paper.

Make

1. Brush salmon with olive oil and season with all-purpose Caribbean blend, salt, and pepper.
2. Mix together pumpkin seeds and sesame seeds in a shallow dish.
3. Press salmon, flesh-side down, into the seeds, and place face-up on the baking pan. Repeat with all filets.
4. Bake in the oven until salmon is cooked through, about 20 minutes. Time will depend on thickness of filets.

Appendix C
Cancer Nutrition Myths

In a world filled with endless health advice, it's easy to get swept up in popular ideas about food and cancer. But many of these "truths" are based on myths rather than solid science, which can lead to confusion and even unhelpful dietary choices.

In this appendix, we'll tackle the top five cancer nutrition myths, focusing on how each relates to a BLOCK pillar. By understanding these myths, you'll be better equipped to make choices that truly protect and support your body's defenses.

Myth Busters

Myth #1

Sugar "feeds" cancer, so cutting it out completely will prevent cancer.

- **Reality:** While cancer cells consume more glucose (sugar) than normal cells, there's no direct evidence that eating sugar causes cancer to develop. All cells, including healthy ones, need glucose for energy. The key is to avoid excessive sugar intake, which can lead to weight gain—a known risk factor for several cancers. Focusing on a balanced diet that limits added sugars supports overall health without "feeding" cancer cells any more than it fuels other cells.
- **Takeaway:** Instead of avoiding all sugar, focus on limiting added sugars and choose whole fruits and nutrient-dense foods for natural sweetness. Think of sugar like paint on your house: a small amount completes the look, but too much can clog and damage the protective layer.

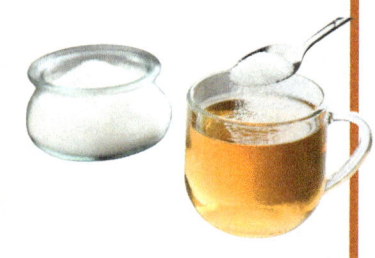

Myth #2

Eating "superfoods" alone can prevent cancer.
- **Reality:** While certain nutrient-rich foods like berries, leafy greens, soursop, moringa, and turmeric are packed with beneficial compounds, no single food alone can prevent cancer. A balanced diet rich in a variety of nutrients is more effective for overall cancer prevention than relying on specific "superfoods." Cancer prevention is about a holistic approach that combines balanced nutrition with other healthy lifestyle choices.
- **Takeaway:** Include a variety of nutritious foods rather than relying on one or two "superfoods". It's like fire prevention: while water is essential, you need multiple resources—like fire alarms, extinguishers, and firefighters—to fully protect the house.

Myth #3

You should avoid soy if you have a strong family history of breast cancer.
- **Reality:** Soy contains phytoestrogens, plant compounds that resemble estrogen but act differently in the body. Studies show that moderate consumption of whole soy foods (like tofu, edamame, and soy milk) does not increase cancer risk, even for those with a family history of breast cancer. In fact, soy may have protective benefits due to its support for cellular repair and overall health.
- **Takeaway:** Whole soy foods can be safely included in a balanced diet, even with a family history of breast cancer. Avoid heavily processed soy products, which may lack the same benefits. Soy is like a skilled repair worker for your body—it has the tools to support your cells, but it works best when it's part of a balanced team (your entire diet).

Myth #4

Acidic foods increase cancer risk by making your body more acidic.

- **Reality:** The body regulates its pH levels tightly, regardless of the foods you consume. While certain acidic foods (like citrus or tomatoes) may seem to affect pH, they don't alter the body's overall acidity in a way that impacts cancer risk. An "alkaline diet" can be healthy because it encourages plant-based foods, but it's the balance of nutrients—not acidity—that truly matters for cancer prevention.
- **Takeaway:** Enjoy a variety of plant-based foods without worrying about acidity. Your immune system functions like a well-calibrated security system—it doesn't depend on your diet's pH level but on a steady supply of diverse, balanced nutrients to stay alert and ready to protect.

Myth #5

Avoiding all fats will reduce your cancer risk.

- **Reality:** While it's beneficial to limit unhealthy fats (like trans fats and excessive saturated fats), healthy fats from sources like olive oil, nuts, seeds, and fatty fish are essential for cellular health and may even help reduce inflammation. Instead of avoiding fats altogether, focus on including healthy fats in your diet, which supports your body's natural "cleaning" systems by maintaining efficient function and reducing cancer risk.
- **Takeaway:** Include healthy fats like avocados, nuts, seeds, and fish in your diet. It's like keeping the plumbing in good shape—healthy fats keep everything flowing smoothly, while unhealthy fats can clog the system and create blockages.

Myth Busters

Appendix D

Nutrition Boosters Guide

This guide offers practical tips for integrating the top nutritional boosters—turmeric, green tea, garlic, omega-3s, and ginger—into your daily routine. These boosters are listed in the order of how strongly they support your health, starting with those that offer the most overall benefits. Each booster includes safe daily dosages, recommended timing, available forms, and easy incorporation methods. While these are the top boosters for cancer reduction, others, like soursop, moringa, noni, and baobab, also provide valuable health benefits. Be sure to consult a healthcare provider before introducing new supplements, particularly if you have health conditions or are on medications.

Practical Tips

- **Meal Plan:** Choose recipes that naturally include these boosters to streamline integration.
- **Smoothie Boosters:** Add turmeric, ginger, green tea (matcha powder), or omega-3 supplements (like flax or chia seeds) to morning smoothies.
- **Routine Habits:** Make ginger or green tea a morning staple, while garlic and turmeric can be regular additions to lunch and dinner.
- **Supplementing Wisely**: Select supplements if fresh or powdered forms aren't convenient, particularly for curcumin and fish oil, which are more effective in concentrated forms.

With these practical tips, you're equipped to make each nutritional booster a seamless part of your daily routine. As you move forward, explore each supplement in detail on the following pages, and discover how these versatile additions can strengthen your health journey.

Turmeric

Turmeric, a golden-yellow root native to Southeast Asia, has been used in Ayurvedic and traditional Chinese medicine for thousands of years. Known as "Indian saffron," it contains curcumin, which gives turmeric its color and a long-standing role in natural healing.

Dosage & Tips

- **Daily Dosage:** 500-1,000 mg of curcumin extract daily, divided into two doses (about 1/4 to 1/2 teaspoon turmeric powder daily).
- **Timing:** Take with meals for better absorption, ideally with a healthy fat source to enhance bioavailability.
- **Forms Available:** Fresh root, dried powder, capsules, or curcumin extract supplements.

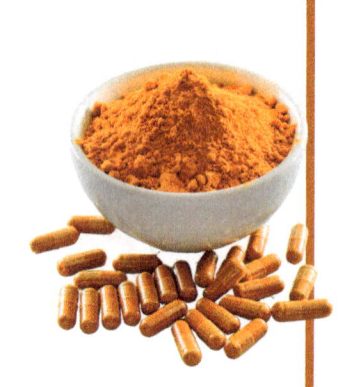

Ways to Incorporate

- **Tea:** Brew turmeric tea by steeping a teaspoon of turmeric powder or fresh turmeric in hot water, adding a dash of black pepper and honey for flavor.
- **Meals:** Add turmeric powder to soups, curries, and stews, or mix into salad dressings.
- **Smoothies:** Blend fresh turmeric or powdered form into smoothies with coconut oil for better absorption.
- **Supplements:** For more potent, consistent doses, consider a curcumin supplement with piperine (black pepper extract) for enhanced absorption.

Green Tea

Green tea, originally from China, is made from the unoxidized leaves of the Camellia sinensis plant. Valued for thousands of years, it's rich in catechins and antioxidants like EGCG and has long been used in traditional medicine for its calming and restorative effects.

Dosage & Tips

- **Daily Dosage:** 3-4 cups of brewed green tea or 300-400 mg of green tea extract.
- **Timing:** Spread throughout the day, ideally before meals for optimal absorption and to manage caffeine sensitivity.
- **Forms Available:** Loose leaves, tea bags, extract capsules, or matcha powder (all available in decaf versions).

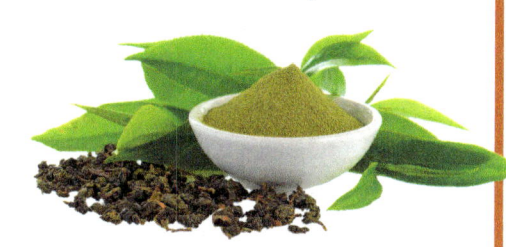

Ways to Incorporate

- **Tea:** Enjoy green tea hot or iced, aiming for a cup before meals or as a refreshing mid-morning or afternoon beverage.
- **Matcha Powder:** Add matcha powder to smoothies, oatmeal, or yogurt for a concentrated dose of EGCG.
- **In Cooking:** Use green tea as a cooking liquid for rice or grains to infuse flavor and add antioxidants.
- **Supplements:** If brewing tea isn't convenient, opt for green tea extract capsules standardized for EGCG content.

Garlic

Garlic, a plant in the onion family, has been valued for its medicinal and culinary uses for thousands of years, dating back to ancient Egypt. Known for its strong aroma and pungent flavor, its sulfur-rich compounds make garlic one of the most potent and widely used herbs for health support.

Dosage & Tips

- **Daily Dosage:** 1-2 cloves of fresh garlic or 600-1,200 mg of garlic extract.
- **Timing:** Take with meals to reduce digestive upset.
- **Forms Available:** Fresh cloves, garlic powder, aged garlic extract, or odor-free capsules.

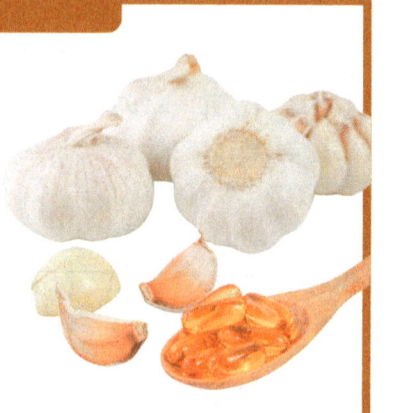

Ways to Incorporate

- **Raw:** For stronger effects, crush or mince raw garlic and let sit for 10 minutes before using to activate beneficial compounds.
- **Cooking:** Use raw garlic in sauces, marinades, and salad dressings, or add to stir-fries and roasted vegetables.
- **In Soups and Broths:** Add fresh garlic during the final cooking stages of soups or broths to retain its active compounds.
- **Supplements:** Choose aged garlic extract for a gentler form that retains health benefits with less pungency.

Omega-3

Omega-3 fatty acids are essential fats primarily found in fish and some plants. Known as "good fats," they were first noted for their health benefits among the Inuit population of Greenland, who consumed large amounts of fish and exhibited heart health benefits linked to these fats.

Dosage & Tips

- **Daily Dosage:** 1,000-2,000 mg of combined EPA and DHA from fish oil or algae oil.
- **Timing:** Take with meals for better absorption and to minimize any aftertaste.
- **Forms Available:** Softgel capsules, liquid fish oil, algae oil (for a plant-based option), or natural sources from fatty fish.

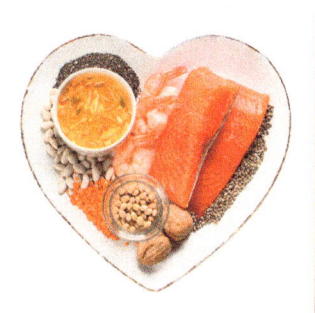

Ways to Incorporate

- **Meals:** Include 2-3 servings of fatty fish like salmon, sardines, herring, or mackerel per week for a natural omega-3 source (EPA and DHA). For a plant-based omega-3 source (ALA), add chia seeds, walnuts, or flaxseeds in cereals, salads, and snacks.
- **Smoothies:** Add a teaspoon of lemon-flavored liquid fish oil or algae oil to smoothies to mask any aftertaste.
- **Supplements:** Choose high-quality fish oil or algae oil supplements certified for purity, containing both EPA and DHA.

Ginger

Ginger, a flowering plant native to Southeast Asia, has a root that's been used as both a spice and medicine for thousands of years. Highly valued in Ayurvedic and Chinese medicine, its peppery, slightly sweet flavor enhances culinary dishes and supports traditional healing practices.

Dosage & Tips

- **Daily Dosage:** 1-2 grams of ginger powder or fresh ginger, or up to 500 mg of ginger extract capsules.
- **Timing:** Anytime, though it can be particularly helpful before meals to aid digestion.
- **Forms Available:** Fresh root, dried powder, crystallized, extract capsules, or tea.

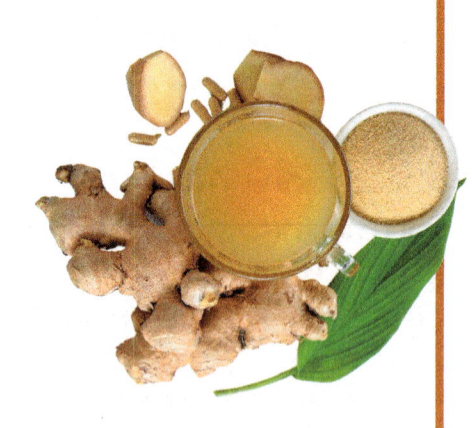

Ways to Incorporate

- **Tea:** Brew ginger tea by simmering fresh ginger slices in hot water. Add honey or lemon for flavor.
- **In Cooking:** Use fresh or powdered ginger in stir-fries, marinades, and curries for flavor and health benefits.
- **Smoothies and Juices:** Blend fresh ginger with other fruits and vegetables for a refreshing, spicy kick.
- **Supplements:** Opt for ginger extract capsules for convenience, especially if using ginger for anti-inflammatory benefits.

Appendix E
Healthy Swap Guide

This guide offers healthier swaps for everyday foods, aligning with the BLOCK pillars to help build a foundation that resists cancer. Each option replaces processed ingredients and refined sugars with nutrient-rich choices, creating stronger, more nourishing meals.

Sugary Beverages

- **Swap:** Soda, sweetened juice, and energy drinks
- **Alternative:** Infused water with fruit slices (e.g., berries, cucumber, lemon, lime, mango, or starfruit)
  - **Why It's Better:** Provides hydration without added sugars, and fruit infusions add natural antioxidants and vitamins.
- **Alternative:** Coconut water (unsweetened)
  - **Why It's Better:** Coconut water has electrolytes and natural sugars, offering a healthier hydration boost.

Processed Meats

- **Swap:** Bacon, sausage, and deli meats
- **Alternative:** Grilled or baked chicken breast, turkey, or local fresh-caught fish
  - **Why It's Better:** Lower in saturated fats and sodium, reducing cancer risk associated with processed meats.
- **Alternative:** Beans and legumes (e.g., black-eyed peas, lentils, pigeon peas, or red beans) in soups and salads
  - **Why It's Better:** Plant-based proteins offer fiber, antioxidants, and fewer processed additives.

Healthy Swap Guide, cont.

Fried Foods

- **Swap:** French fries, fried chicken, and potato chips
- **Alternative:** Baked or air-fried sweet potato wedges
  - **Why It's Better:** Sweet potatoes provide fiber, vitamin A, and fewer unhealthy fats compared to fried options.
- **Alternative:** Baked plantains or taro root chips
  - **Why It's Better:** Plantains are rich in potassium and provide a lower-fat option with fiber and vitamins.

Refined Grains

- **Swap:** White rice, white bread, and refined pasta
- **Alternative:** Quinoa, brown rice, or farro
  - **Why It's Better:** Whole grains are rich in fiber and essential nutrients, supporting digestion and reducing cancer risk.
- **Alternative:** Whole-grain bread or cassava flour bread
  - **Why It's Better:** Whole-grain bread contains fiber and B vitamins, while cassava flour is gluten-free and provides more nutrients than refined flour.

Refined Cooking Oils

- **Swap:** Vegetable oil, corn oil, and shortening
- **Alternative:** Extra-virgin olive oil or avocado oil
  - **Why It's Better:** Both oils are high in monounsaturated fats, supporting heart health and reducing inflammation.

Healthy Swap Guide, cont.

High-Calorie Condiments

- **Swap:** Mayonnaise, creamy dressings, and sugary sauces
- **Alternative:** Avocado or hummus as spreads
  - **Why It's Better:** Both are nutrient-rich and provide healthy fats and fiber, supporting cell health and reducing inflammation.
- **Alternative:** Olive oil and balsamic vinegar for salads
  - **Why It's Better:** Olive oil is packed with healthy fats and antioxidants, while balsamic vinegar adds flavor without added sugars.

Sugary Snacks & Desserts

- **Swap:** Candy, cookies, and pastries
- **Alternative:** Fresh fruit, such as papaya, soursop, or guava, with a sprinkle of coconut flakes
  - **Why It's Better:** Fruits add natural sweetness, fiber, and antioxidants without added sugars.
- **Alternative:** Dark chocolate (70% or higher cocoa content)
  - **Why It's Better:** Dark chocolate has antioxidants and less sugar than milk chocolate and most sweets.

These healthy swaps support the BLOCK pillars by cutting down on processed ingredients and adding more antioxidants, anti-inflammatory, and digestion-supporting nutrients. With small, steady changes, you can strengthen your body's defenses and enjoy a balanced, nourishing diet.

Appendix F
Hydration Essentials

Keeping your body hydrated is key for smooth functioning, helping maintain energy, focus, digestion, and even mood. While thirst is a natural reminder to drink, it often comes too late—if you feel thirsty, you're likely already dehydrated. This is especially true in air-conditioned spaces or for older adults, as thirst signals may be weaker. Here's a quick guide to the stages of dehydration, signs to watch for, and why it's essential to sip water regularly, even if you're not feeling thirsty.

Dehydration Stages

Mild Dehydration:
- **Signs:** Dry mouth, mild headache, slight fatigue, and reduced focus.
- **Solution:** Drink water steadily throughout the day, aiming for 8–10 cups to prevent dehydration.

Moderate Dehydration:
- **Signs:** Dizziness, darker urine, dry skin, and more fatigue.
- **Solution:** Add hydrating drinks like coconut water and include foods like watermelon.

Severe Dehydration:
- **Signs:** Confusion, rapid heartbeat, and extreme tiredness.
- **Solution:** Seek medical care immediately, as severe dehydration requires quick rehydration.

Hydration helps the body remove waste, keeps tiredness away, and maintains steady energy. Drinking water regularly—even before you feel thirsty—keeps your body in balance, helps your organs function smoothly, and supports overall health.

Hydration Essentials, cont.

Hydration Recommendations

- **Start the Day with Water:** Drink room-temperature or warm water first thing in the morning to boost your metabolism, help with digestion, and flush out waste.
- **Drink Before Meals:** Having a glass of water about 15-30 minutes before eating can improve digestion and help your body absorb nutrients.
- **Stay Hydrated During Exercise:** Drink more water when physically active. Try coconut water or herbal teas for added hydration and electrolytes.

Hydrating Snacks

Enjoy these everyday snacks for a refreshing way to stay hydrated and get essential nutrients. Try to have these water-rich snacks a few times each day to keep your body well-supported.

- Apples
- Bell peppers
- Blackberries
- Blueberries
- Cantaloupes
- Carambolas (starfruits)
- Celery
- Cherries
- Coconut water
- Cucumbers
- Grapefruits
- Grapes
- Guavas
- Honeydew melons
- Kiwis
- Mangoes
- Oranges
- Papayas
- Peaches
- Pineapples
- Raspberries
- Strawberries
- Tomatoes
- Watermelons

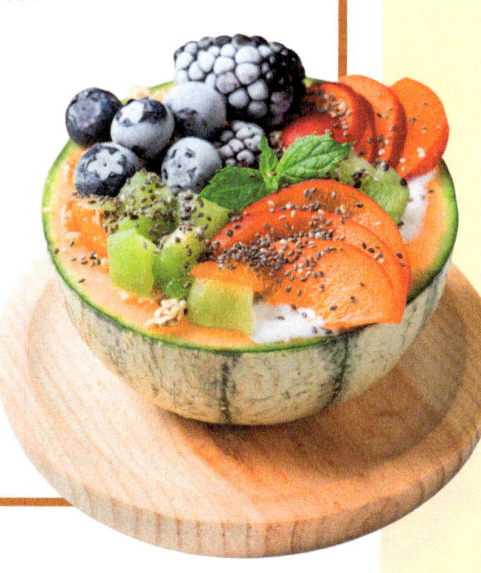

Refresh & Replenish

Hydration Essentials, cont.

These hydration recipes offer simple, flavorful ways to boost your water intake while adding essential electrolytes like potassium, magnesium, and sodium. Store in the refrigerator for up to 24 hours and enjoy these refreshing drinks to stay energized all day.

Watermelon Refresher

Ingredients
- 1 quart (4 cups) water
- 2 cups diced fresh watermelon
- 1/8 tsp Celtic sea salt

Instructions
Blend the watermelon with water until smooth. Add the sea salt, stir, and serve over ice.

Chia Seed Water

Ingredients
- 1 quart (4 cups) water
- 2 Tbsp chia seeds
- 1 Tbsp lemon or lime (optional)

Instructions
Mix chia seeds with water and let it sit for 10-15 minutes until the seeds swell. Add lemon or lime juice for flavor if desired, stir well, and serve.

Celery & Cucumber Mix

Ingredients
- 1 quart (4 cups) water
- 1 cucumber, chopped
- 2 celery stalks, chopped
- 1/8 tsp Himalayan salt

Instructions
Blend cucumber, celery, and water until smooth. Strain the mixture, add sea salt, stir well, and serve chilled.

ACV Vitality Tonic

Ingredients
- 1 quart (4 cups) water
- 2 tsp apple cider vinegar
- 1/8 tsp Celtic sea salt
- 1 tsp honey (optional)

Instructions
Mix all ingredients in a pitcher, stir well, and enjoy.

Hydration Essentials, cont.

Citrus Replenisher

Ingredients

- 1 quart (4 cups) water
- Juice of 1 lemon or lime
- Juice of 1/2 orange
- 1/8 tsp Himalayan salt
- 1 tsp honey (optional)

Instructions

Mix all ingredients in a pitcher, stir well, and serve over ice.

Aloe Vera Elixir

Ingredients

- 1 quart (4 cups) water
- 1/4 cup aloe vera gel (fresh or store-bought)
- 1 Tbsp lemon or lime
- 1 tsp honey (optional)

Instructions

Blend the aloe vera gel with water and lime juice until smooth. Add honey if desired, stir, and serve over ice.

Herbal Infusion

Ingredients

- 1 quart (4 cups) water
- 2 Tbsp dried dandelion or nettle leaves

Instructions

Steep the leaves in boiling water for 10-15 minutes. Strain and cool. Serve over ice or refrigerate for later.

Leafy Green Water

Ingredients

- 1 quart (4 cups) water
- 1/2 cup spinach or kale

Instructions

Blend spinach or kale with water until smooth. Strain, and serve over ice.

Remember, hydration boosts energy, helps digestion, and supports overall health. Use these tips and recipes to make it a simple daily habit.

Hydration Recipes

Appendix G
Stress-Relief Practices

Chronic stress can lead to inflammation, increasing health risks over time. Try these simple techniques to ease stress and lower inflammation. Practicing them regularly can boost your endurance and support the BLOCK pillars.

While you can do these techniques anywhere, a quiet space free of distractions—like a calm corner at home, a comfortable spot in nature, or even a quiet area at work—can help you focus better and make each practice more effective and rejuvenating.

Techniques

Deep Breathing
- **How-to:** Breathe deeply through your nose, allowing your belly to expand. Exhale slowly through your mouth. Repeat for 1–2 minutes.
- **Benefit:** Calms the nervous system, reduces stress, and lowers inflammation.

Guided Imagery
- **How-to:** Close your eyes and imagine a peaceful scene—perhaps a beach or forest. Visualize yourself in that place, taking in the sights, sounds, and smells for 3–5 minutes.
- **Benefit:** Reduces tension, helps shift focus away from stressors, and encourages relaxation.

Progressive Muscle Relaxation
- **How-to:** Starting with your toes, tense each muscle group for 5 seconds, then relax. Gradually move up the body to release tension throughout.
- **Benefit:** Relieves physical tension from stress, promoting a sense of overall relaxation.

Stress-Relief Practices, cont.

Techniques, cont.

5-Minute Walk or Stretch
- **How-to:** Take a slow walk or stretch gently, focusing on breathing and the rhythm of movement.
- **Benefit:** Physical movement releases endorphins, which help to reduce stress hormones and inflammation.

Mindful Breathing Exercise
- **How-to:** Breathe in for a count of 4, hold for 4, exhale for 4, hold again for 4. Repeat several times.
- **Benefit:** This "box breathing" method eases anxiety, improves focus, and helps balance mood.

Journaling
- **How-to:** Spend 5 minutes writing down your thoughts, concerns, or positive affirmations.
- **Benefit:** Helps release mental tension and supports positive thinking, reducing the effects of stress.

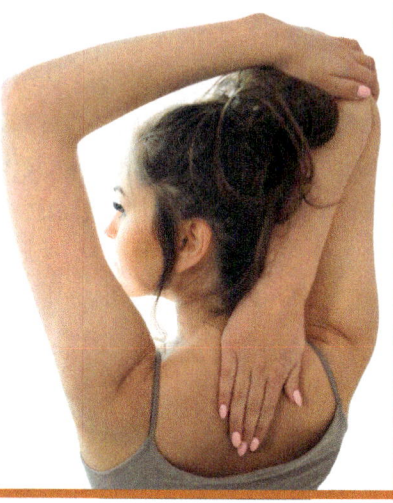

You can practice these techniques at home, at work, or on the go to manage stress and support a balanced, healthy body. Whether it's taking a few deep breaths during a busy day or relaxing quietly before bed, these practices help keep you grounded and calm. Creating a routine and trying different techniques can show what works best, making stress relief a natural part of your daily life and a strong support for each BLOCK pillar.

Appendix H
Sleep Hygiene Tips

Restful Sleep Setup

- **Limit Screen Time:** Power down electronic devices at least one hour before bed. Blue light from screens can disrupt melatonin production, making it harder to fall asleep.
- **Set a Consistent Sleep Schedule:** Go to bed and wake up at the same time each day, even on weekends. This routine helps regulate your body's internal clock.
- **Create a Comfortable Bedroom:** Keep your sleep space cool, dark, and quiet. Use blackout curtains, earplugs, or white noise machines if needed to minimize disruptions.
- **Choose Relaxing Activities Before Bed:** Opt for quiet, calming activities such as reading a book, listening to soft music, or practicing gentle stretches.

Wind-Down Routine

- **Dim the Lights:** Start lowering the lights around you 30 minutes before bed to cue your body that it's time to wind down.
- **Practice Deep Breathing:** Try 5-10 minutes of slow, deep breathing exercises. This can calm the nervous system, preparing your body for rest.
- **Jot Down Thoughts:** Keep a journal by your bed to write down any lingering thoughts or worries. This can help clear your mind and relieve stress before sleeping.
- **Have a Cup of Herbal Tea:** Sip on a caffeine-free tea, like chamomile, soursop, or valerian root, as part of your bedtime routine.

Appendix I
Weekly Exercise Guide

Getting Started

Regular physical activity is a key component in reinforcing each BLOCK pillar, strengthening your body's defenses, and promoting overall wellness. This sample weekly exercise guide includes a balanced mix of cardio, strength, flexibility, and balance exercises to support your fitness journey. For those new to exercise, a few beginner-friendly tips and reminders about the health benefits are also provided.

Sample Weekly Exercise Guide:
- **Cardio (150-200 minutes per week, 3-4 times per week):** Activities like brisk walking, cycling, or dancing to improve heart health and stamina.
- **Strength Training (60-90 minutes per week, 2-3 times per week):** Exercises such as bodyweight exercises, resistance bands, or weight lifting to build muscle and enhance bone density.
- **Flexibility & Balance (30-60 minutes per week, 2-3 times per week):** Gentle stretching, yoga, or Pilates to improve range of motion and reduce injury risk.

Tips for Making Exercise Enjoyable:
- Choose activities you enjoy, like dancing, hiking, or a favorite sport, to stay motivated.
- Incorporate variety into your workouts to keep things interesting and target different muscle groups.
- Consider joining a class or working out with a friend to make it social and engaging.

Exercise for Health

Weekly Exercise Guide, cont.

Safety Tips

If you're new to exercise or have any health conditions, it's important to check if you're ready for physical activity. The Physical Activity Readiness Questionnaire (PAR-Q) below can help spot any possible concerns:

- Has your doctor ever told you to limit physical activity due to a heart condition?
- Do you get chest pain during physical activity?
- Have you had chest pain in the last month unrelated to exercise?
- Do you sometimes lose balance because of dizziness or have you ever lost consciousness?
- Do you have any bone or joint issues that could get worse with physical activity?
- Are you taking medication for blood pressure or a heart condition?
- Is there any other reason you should avoid physical activity?

If you answered "yes" to any of these questions, talk to a healthcare provider before starting a new exercise program. They can give you advice so you can begin safely and build confidence as you go.

With a balanced routine and activities you enjoy, regular exercise can become a lifelong habit, strengthening your body, enhancing your mood, and supporting each BLOCK pillar. Listen to your body, stay consistent, and remember: every step builds a healthier foundation.

Appendix J
Quit Smoking Support

Support Resources

- **National Quitline:** Call 1-800-QUIT-NOW for free support and access to a trained counselor. This service offers personalized guidance, tips, and strategies to help you quit.
- **Smokefree.gov:** Visit Smokefree.gov for online tools, resources, and community support. They offer specific programs for different groups, including veterans, teens, and women.
- **Quit Smoking Apps:** Download the QuitGuide or QuitSTART apps, both designed to help track progress, manage cravings, and provide daily encouragement. Available for free on iOS and Android.
- **American Cancer Society:** Explore resources at cancer.org, including a guide to quitting smoking, support networks, and options for medication assistance.

Health Benefits Over Time

- **20 Minutes After Quitting:** Heart rate and blood pressure begin to drop to healthier levels.
- **12 Hours After Quitting:** Carbon monoxide levels in the blood return to normal, improving oxygen levels.
- **1 to 9 Months After Quitting:** Coughing and shortness of breath decrease as lung function improves.
- **1 Year After Quitting:** Risk of coronary heart disease is half that of a smoker's.
- **5 Years After Quitting:** Risk of mouth, throat, esophagus, and bladder cancer is cut in half.

Appendix K

BLOCK Pillar Plan

This BLOCK Pillar Plan provides a simple daily guide to support each pillar with balanced foods, key supplements, hydration, and healthy habits. By following these steps, you can strengthen your body's natural defenses and create a lasting foundation for overall health and wellness.

BLOCK Pillar Plan

6:30 AM – Wake Up and Hydrate
- 1 glass of water with lemon to rehydrate after sleep
- **Stress Relief:** Start the day with 5 minutes of deep breathing or a light stretching session
- **Weight Awareness:** Morning is the best time to weigh yourself if you are working toward a weight loss or management goal

7:00 AM – Breakfast
- Smoothie: 1 cup spinach (leafy greens), 1 cup mixed berries (berries), 2 Tbsp chia seeds (nuts & seeds), 1 1/2 cups soy milk, and 1/4 tsp fresh turmeric (or 500 mg turmeric supplement)
- Beverage: 1 cup green tea (or 300 mg green tea extract)

9:00 AM – Mid-Morning Hydration
- 1 cup coconut water for hydration and electrolytes

10:00 AM – Morning Snack
- 1/4 cup walnuts (nuts & seeds) and a medium apple
- **Environmental Awareness:** Open a window or add an air-purifying plant to promote cleaner indoor air

12:30 PM – Lunch
- Stir-fry: 1 1/2 cups broccoli (cruciferous), 1 cup chickpeas (beans & legumes), 1 1/2 Tbsp olive oil, and garlic (or 600–1,200 mg garlic supplement)
- Beverage: 1 cup water

BLOCK Pillar Guide, cont.

BLOCK Pillar Plan, cont.

3:00 PM - Mid-Afternoon Hydration
- 1 cup water with a hint of ginger (or 1-2 grams ginger supplement)

3:30 PM - Afternoon Snack
- 1 cup Greek yogurt (plain, non-fat) with 1 Tbsp honey and 1/2 cup blueberries (berries)

4:30 PM - Exercise
- 30 minutes of moderate-intensity activity, such as brisk walking or light jogging
- **Sun Exposure Awareness:** If exercising outdoors, apply SPF 30+ sunscreen for skin protection

6:00 PM - Dinner
- Grilled salmon (5 oz, for omega-3s) with a side of 1 1/2 cups roasted Brussels sprouts (cruciferous) and 1 cup quinoa
- Optional: 1,000 mg omega-3 supplement (EPA/DHA combined) if salmon isn't included in the meal
- Beverage: 1 glass of water

8:30 PM - Evening Wind-Down
- Herbal or soursop tea with ginger (or 1-2 grams ginger supplement) for relaxation and digestion (optional)
- **Stress Relief:** Wrap up the day with 10 minutes of journaling or a few rounds of deep breathing

10:00 PM - Sleep
- Aim for 7-9 hours of restful sleep to support body repair and recovery

Smoke-Free Reminder: Avoid smoking or being around secondhand smoke to keep your body healthy

Health Screening & Genetic Awareness: Schedule recommended health screenings or genetic consultations as part of a proactive approach to cancer prevention

Appendix L

Cancer Resources

This list includes trusted links to organizations, websites, and books with helpful information on cancer prevention, nutrition, and healthy living. You'll find up-to-date research, practical tips, and expert advice to help you make informed health choices. Whether you want to learn more, connect with supportive communities, or find reliable sources, these recommendations can guide you.

Organizations & Websites

National Cancer Institute (NCI)
https://www.cancer.gov
Offers comprehensive information on cancer research, prevention, and treatment from a government-backed perspective.

American Cancer Society (ACS)
https://www.cancer.org
Provides a wide array of resources on cancer types, preventive care, support, and educational materials.

American Institute for Cancer Research (AICR)
https://www.aicr.org
Known for cancer prevention research and resources, especially those centered around diet and lifestyle.

MD Anderson Cancer Center
https://www.mdanderson.org
Provides in-depth information on various cancers and offers resources on treatment options, support services, and lifestyle changes.

Cancer Resources, cont.

Organizations & Websites, cont.

Oncology Nutrition (Academy of Nutrition and Dietetics)
https://www.oncologynutrition.org
Focused on nutrition's role in cancer prevention, treatment, and survivorship, with practical dietary resources and recipes.

The Environmental Working Group (EWG) – Guide to Pesticides in Produce
https://www.ewg.org/foodnews/
A practical resource for identifying pesticide levels in produce, to help people make informed choices about fruits and vegetables.

Memorial Sloan Kettering Cancer Center – About Herbs, Botanicals & Other Products
https://www.mskcc.org/cancer-care/diagnosis-treatment/symptom-management/integrative-medicine/herbs
Details various herbs and supplements, providing evidence-based information about their potential benefits and risks for cancer patients.

National Center for Complementary and Integrative Health (NCCIH)
https://www.nccih.nih.gov
Provides research-based insights on complementary therapies, including those that may support cancer prevention and treatment.

Resources & Support

Cancer Resources, cont.

Books

"Anticancer: A New Way of Life" by David Servan-Schreiber, MD, PhD
Focuses on the holistic approach to cancer prevention and treatment through lifestyle changes, backed by scientific research.

"The Cancer-Fighting Kitchen: Nourishing, Big-Flavor Recipes for Cancer Treatment and Recovery" by Rebecca Katz
Offers a guide to nutritious and palatable recipes tailored to help patients during and after cancer treatment.

"How to Prevent and Treat Cancer with Natural Medicine" by Michael Murray, ND, et al.
Combines insights from naturopathic and conventional medicine to offer natural ways of supporting cancer prevention and care.

"Radical Remission: Surviving Cancer Against All Odds" by Kelly A. Turner, PhD
Based on research of cancer survivors who defied medical predictions, this book explores nine factors that could help improve recovery and survival.

"The Spectrum: A Scientifically Proven Program to Feel Better, Live Longer, Lose Weight, and Gain Health" by Dean Ornish, MD
Outlines a flexible and comprehensive approach to health improvement, covering nutrition, exercise, stress management, and lifestyle adjustments to support both prevention and recovery from chronic conditions, including cancer.

References

- Aggarwal, B. B., & Harikumar, K. B. (2009). Potential therapeutic effects of curcumin, the anti-inflammatory agent, against cancer, cardiovascular, pulmonary, and autoimmune diseases. International Journal of Biochemistry & Cell Biology, 41(1), 40-59. https://doi.org/10.1016/j.biocel.2008.06.010
- American Cancer Society. (2022). Cancer prevention and early detection. https://www.cancer.org/healthy.html
- American Cancer Society. (2020). Skin cancer prevention and early detection. https://www.cancer.org
- American Institute for Cancer Research. (2021). Healthy recipes and food choices to prevent cancer. https://www.aicr.org/cancer-prevention/food-facts/
- Beliveau, R., & Gingras, D. (2006). Foods that fight cancer: Preventing cancer through diet. DK Publishing.
- Conlon, M. A., & Bird, A. R. (2015). The impact of diet and lifestyle on gut microbiota and human health. Nutrients, 7(1), 17-44. https://doi.org/10.3390/nu7010017
- Couzin-Frankel, J. (2013). Cancer immunotherapy. Science, 342(6165), 1432-1433. https://doi.org/10.1126/science.342.6165.1432
- Halliwell, B. (2012). Free radicals and antioxidants: Updating a personal view. Nutrition ReviewInternational Agency for Research on Cancer. (2018). IARC monographs on the evaluation of carcinogenic risks to humans: Volume 123. https://monographs.iarc.frs, 70(5), 257-265. https://doi.org/10.1111/j.1753-4887.2012.00476.x
- Harvard T.H. Chan School of Public Health. (n.d.). The Nutrition Source: Healthy eating plate & healthy eating pyramid. https://www.hsph.harvard.edu/nutritionsource/healthy-eating-plate/
- International Agency for Research on Cancer. (2018). IARC monographs on the evaluation of carcinogenic risks to humans: Volume 123.. https://monographs.iarc.fr
- Katz, R. (2017). The cancer-fighting kitchen: Nourishing, big-flavor recipes for cancer treatment and recovery (2nd ed.). Ten Speed Press.
- Larsson, S. C., Kumlin, M., Ingelman-Sundberg, M., & Wolk, A. (2004). Dietary long-chain n-3 fatty acids for the prevention of cancer: A review of potential mechanisms. American Journal of Clinical Nutrition, 79(6), 935-945. https://doi.org/10.1093/ajcn/79.6.935

References, cont.

- Liu, R. H. (2013). Health benefits of fruit and vegetables are from additive and synergistic combinations of phytochemicals. American Journal of Clinical Nutrition, 78(3), 517S-520S. https://doi.org/10.1093/ajcn/78.3.517S
- Lynch, S. V., & Pedersen, O. (2016). The human intestinal microbiome in health and disease. New England Journal of Medicine, 375(24), 2369-2379. https://doi.org/10.1056/NEJMra1600266
- Milner, J. A. (2001). A historical perspective on garlic and cancer. Journal of Nutrition, 131(3), 1027S-1031S. https://doi.org/10.1093/jn/131.3.1027S
- National Cancer Institute. (2021). Cancer information and resources. https://www.cancer.gov/about-cancer/causes-prevention
- National Center for Complementary and Integrative Health. (2021). Relaxation techniques for health. https://www.nccih.nih.gov/health/relaxation-techniques-for-health
- National Cancer Institute. (2018). BRCA mutations: Cancer risk and genetic testing. https://www.cancer.gov/about-cancer/causes-prevention/genetics/brca-fact-sheet
- Ornish, D. (2007). The spectrum: A scientifically proven program to feel better, live longer, lose weight, and gain health. Ballantine Books.
- Sharifi-Rad, J., El Rayess, Y., Abi Rizk, A., Sadaka, C., Zgheib, R., Zam, W., Sestito, S., Rapposelli, S., Neffe-Skocińska, K., Zielińska, D., Salehi, B., Setzer, W. N., Dosoky, N. S., Taheri, Y., El Beyrouthy, M., Martorell, M., Ostrander, E. A., Suleria, H. A. R., Cho, W. C., … Martins, N. (2020). Turmeric and its major compound curcumin on health: Bioactive effects and safety profiles for food, pharmaceutical, biotechnological, and medicinal applications. Frontiers in Pharmacology, 11, 01021. https://doi.org/10.3389/fphar.2020.01021
- Shukla, Y., & Singh, M. (2007). Cancer preventive properties of ginger: A brief review. Food and Chemical Toxicology, 45(5), 683-690. https://doi.org/10.1016/j.fct.2006.11.002
- Yang, C. S., & Wang, H. (2016). Cancer preventive activities of tea catechins. Molecules, 21(12), 1679. https://doi.org/10.3390/molecules21121679
- Zauber, A. G. (2015). The impact of screening on colorectal cancer mortality and incidence—has it really made a difference? Digestive Diseases and Sciences, 60(3), 681–691. doi:10.1007/s10620-014-3484-3

Interested in learning more?

Let's Connect

- preventionspecialists.usvi
- @preventionspecialists.vi
- @preventionspecialists.usvi
- @thepreventionspecialists6852
- www.tpsvi.com
- lhenry@tpsvi.com

Strengthen Your Body from Within— Because the Best Defense Starts with You!

One of the most powerful truths in health and healing is that small, intentional choices add up. Science confirms that while genetics play a role, your daily habits and nutrition have a profound impact on disease prevention. The food you eat, the way you manage stress, and the lifestyle choices you make can either fuel disease or fortify your body's natural defenses.

The choice is yours. Take control, embrace prevention, and BLOCK cancer naturally—one step at a time.

There is one more step we need you to take!

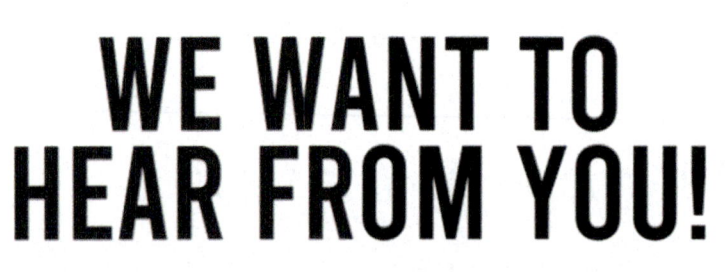

WE WANT TO HEAR FROM YOU!

IF YOU ENJOYED THIS BOOK, PLEASE LEAVE A REVIEW TO HELP OTHERS

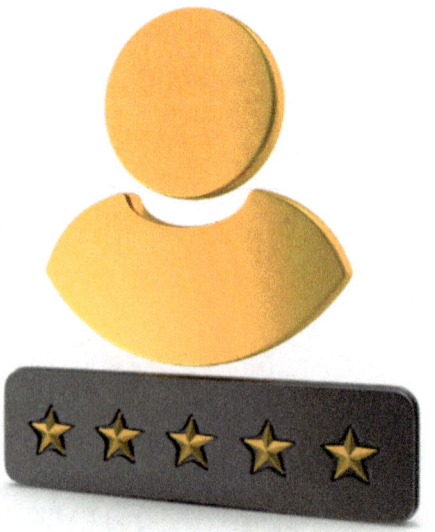

As an author, I deeply value your feedback. Your thoughts help shape future content, ensuring that more people have access to the knowledge and tools they need to live healthier lives. More importantly, your review can help others on their journey to cancer prevention by guiding them toward practical, science-backed solutions.

Scan the QR code to leave your review.

Your health matters. Your voice matters. Thank you for being part of this mission!

Scan to Review

Printed in Great Britain
by Amazon